Lecture Notes on Dermatology

ROBIN GRAHAM-BROWN
BSc, MB, BS (Lond), FRCP
Consultant Dermatologist,
The Leicester Royal Infirmary, Leicester,
and Clinical Teacher (Dermatology),
University of Leicester School of Medicine

TONY BURNS
MB, BS (Lond), FRCP
Consultant Dermatologist,
The Leicester Royal Infirmary, Leicester,
and Clinical Teacher (Dermatology),
University of Leicester School of Medicine

SIXTH EDITION

OXFORD

BLACKWELL SCIENTIFIC PUBLICATIONS

LONDON EDINBURGH BOSTON

MELBOURNE PARIS BERLIN VIENNA

To all medical students and to our children:
James, Matthew, John, Joseph and David

© 1965, 1969, 1973, 1977,
1983, 1990 by
Blackwell Scientific Publications
Editorial Offices:
Osney Mead, Oxford OX2 0EL
25 John Street, London WC1N 2BL
23 Ainslie Place, Edinburgh EH3 6AJ
3 Cambridge Center, Suite 208
  Cambridge, Massachusetts 02142, USA
54 University Street, Carlton
  Victoria 3053, Australia

First published 1965
Reprinted 1966
Second edition 1969
Third edition 1973
Reprinted 1975
Fourth edition 1977
Reprinted 1979, 1981
Fifth edition 1983
Reprinted 1988
Sixth edition 1990

Set by Times Graphics, Singapore
Printed and bound in Hong Kong by
Dah-Hua Printing Press Ltd

DISTRIBUTORS

UK
  Marston Book Services Ltd
  PO Box 87
  Oxford OX2 0DT
  (Orders: Tel. 0865-791155
          Fax: 0865-791927
          Telex: 837515)

USA
  Mosby–Year Book, Inc.
  200 North LaSalle Street
  Chicago, Illinois 60601
  (Orders: Tel: (312) 726-9733)

Canada
  Mosby–Year Book, Inc.
  5240 Finch Avenue East
  Scarborough, Ontario
  (Orders: Tel: (416) 298-1588)

Australia
  Blackwell Scientific Publications
  (Australia) Pty Ltd
  54 University Street
  Carlton, Victoria 3053
  (Orders: Tel: (03) 347-0300)

British Library
Cataloguing in Publication Data

Graham-Brown, R. A. C. (Robin A. C.)
  Lecture notes on dermatology—6th ed.
  I. Title II. Burns, D. Anthony
  III. Solomons, Bethel
  616.5

  ISBN 0-632-02765-7 (BSP)
  ISBN 0-632-028823 (Four Dragons)

Contents

Preface

We are delighted to have been asked to take over the dermatological member of the ever-popular 'Lecture Notes' series. We have started completely from scratch to try and produce a book that is both compact, concise and readable as well as covering what we believe to be the most relevant aspects of modern clinical dermatology.

Our aims in carrying out this revision are exactly the same as those expressed by Dr Bethel Solomons in his preface to the first edition, which appeared in 1965: to provide an introduction to dermatology for medical students and general practitioners. Our approach to the task has been based on the aims and objectives that we set ourselves in teaching dermatology to the medical students who pass through our department in Leicester, i.e. that after the course, the student should:

1 Have some knowledge of the structure and function of the skin.

2 Be able to recognize and initiate treatment for the common skin diseases.

3 Appreciate the importance of some of the rarer and more severe dermatological disorders.

4 Be able to give an adequate account of his or her findings and conclusions to a third party.

We think that achieving these basic objectives will be of practical value both to those studying dermatology as undergraduates and to the doctor dealing with skin disease in a non-specialist setting. We also hope that exposure to 'Lecture Notes on Dermatology', together with clinical examination of patients, will provide a stimulus to some to take a deeper interest in the skin and the problems suffered by those with skin disease.

If we have been successful in achieving these objectives, then we believe that this new-look 'Lecture Notes on Dermatology' will continue to be as popular as its predecessors and companions in the series.

Robin Graham-Brown
Tony Burns

Acknowledgements

We would particularly like to thank Drs Imrich Sarkany and Charles Calnan under whose guidance we have both learned dermatology. We are also grateful to them for some of the illustrations.

We are grateful to our students who remind us constantly of the importance of clarity in communication.

Finally we must thank Peter Saugman who offered us the opportunity to write this book and John Robson, Vicky Murray, and all the staff at Blackwell Scientific Publications, who have helped us patiently through the editing and production stages.

Chapter 1
Structure and Function of the Skin, Hair and Nails

Skin, skin is a wonderful thing,
Keeps the outside out and the inside in.

This, you may consider, is the boring part of the book, but it is essential to have some background knowledge of the normal structure and function of any organ before you can hope to understand the abnormal. Skin is the icing on the anatomical cake, and without it not only would we all look rather unappealing, but a variety of unpleasant physiological phenomena would bring about our demise. You have probably never contemplated your skin a great deal, except in the throes of narcissistic admiration, or when it has been blemished by some disorder, but hopefully by the end of this first chapter you may be persuaded that it really is quite a remarkable organ, and that you are lucky to be on such intimate terms with it.

Skin structure
The skin is composed of two layers, the epidermis and the dermis. The epidermis, which is the outer layer, and its appendages (hair, nails, sebaceous glands and sweat glands) are derived from the embryonic ectoderm. The dermis is of mesodermal origin.

The epidermis
The epidermis is a multilayered structure which renews itself continuously by cell division in its deepest layer—the basal layer. The principal cell type, the epidermal cell, is most commonly referred to as a keratinocyte. The cells produced by cell division in the basal layer constitute the prickle cell layer and as they ascend towards the surface they undergo a process known as keratinization which involves the synthesis of the fibrous protein keratin. A typical cell takes approximately 30 days to pass from the basal layer to the surface of the epidermis (epidermal transit time). The cells on the surface of the skin, forming the horny layer (stratum corneum), are fully keratinized dead cells which are gradually abraded by day to day wear and tear from the environment. If you bathe after a period of several days' deprivation of contact with water (a house without central heating in mid-winter, somewhere in the Northern Hemisphere, is ideal for this experiment) you will notice that as you towel yourself you are rubbing off small balls of keratin—keratin which has built up because of your insanitary habits. When a plaster cast is removed from a limb after several weeks in situ there is usually a thick layer of surface keratin, the removal of which provides hours of absorbing occupational therapy.

1

Look at the layers more closely (Fig. 1.1). The basal layer is composed of columnar cells which are anchored to a basement membrane—this lies between the epidermis and dermis. The basement membrane is a multilayered structure from which anchoring fibrils extend into the superficial dermis. Interspersed amongst the basal cells are melanocytes, large dendritic cells derived from the neural crest, which are responsible for melanin pigment production. Melanocytes contain cytoplasmic organelles called melanosomes in which melanin is synthesized from tyrosine. The enzyme tyrosinase is essential for melanin production—it is reduced in amount or absent in albinism. The melanosomes migrate along the dendrites of the melanocytes and are transferred to the keratinocytes in the prickle cell layer. In fair-skinned Caucasians the melanosomes are grouped together in 'melanosome complexes', and they gradually degenerate as the keratinocytes move towards the surface of the skin. Negro skin contains the same number of melanocytes as that of fair-skinned Caucasians, but the melanosomes are larger, remain separate, and persist throughout the full thickness of the epidermis. The main stimulus to melanin production is ultraviolet (UV) light. Melanin protects the cell nuclei in the epidermis from the harmful effects of UV radiation. A sun tan is a natural protective mechanism, not some God-given cosmetic boon. Skin neoplasia is extremely uncommon in dark-skinned races because their skin is protected from UV damage by large quantities of melanin. Not so the pale, pimply lager-swilling advert for British manhood who dashes onto the beach in Majorca and flash-fries himself to lobster thermidor on day 1 of his annual hols.

The prickle cell layer acquires its name from the spiky appearance produced by intercellular bridges (desmosomes) which connect adjacent cells. Scattered throughout the prickle cell layer are numbers of dendritic cells called Langerhans cells. They are difficult to see with haematoxylin and eosin staining, but can be demonstrated using special stains. Langerhans cells are probably modified macrophages which originate in the bone marrow and migrate to the

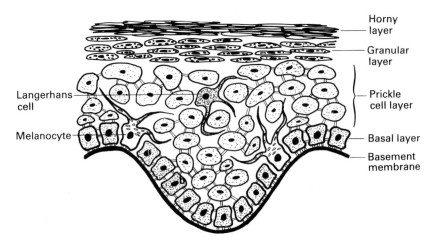

Fig. 1.1. The epidermis.

epidermis. They are the first line of immunological defence against environmental antigens and are responsible for uptake of such antigens and their presentation to immunocompetent lymphocytes, so that an immune response can be mounted.

Above the prickle cell layer is the granular layer which is composed of rather flattened cells containing numerous darkly staining particles known as keratohyalin granules. Also present in the cytoplasm of cells in the granular layer are organelles known as lamellar granules (Odland bodies). Lamellar granules contain lipids and enzymes, and they discharge their contents into the intercelluar spaces between the cells of the granular layer and stratum corneum—providing something akin to 'mortar' between the cellular 'bricks'. In the granular layer the cell membranes become thickened as a result of deposition of dense material on their inner surfaces.

The cells of the stratum corneum are flattened, keratinized cells which are devoid of nuclei and cytoplasmic organelles—these cellular components degenerate in the upper granular layer. Adjacent cells overlap at their margins and this locking together of cells, together with intercellular lipid, forms a very effective barrier. The stratum corneum varies in thickness depending on the region of the body, being thickest over the palms of the hands and soles of the feet.

Keratin production

Keratin is the main structural protein of the epidermis. The keratinocytes in the basal layer and prickle cell layer synthesize keratin filaments (tonofilaments) which aggregate into bundles (tonofibrils). Eventually, in the cells of the stratum corneum, these bundles of keratin filaments form a complex intracellular network embedded in an amorphous protein matrix. This matrix is derived from the keratohyalin granules of the granular layer. Epidermal keratinization results in the production of a barrier which is relatively impermeable to substances passing in or out of the body.

Epidermal appendages

The eccrine and apocrine sweat glands, the hair and sebaceous glands, and the nails, constitute the epidermal appendages.

Eccrine sweat glands

Eccrine sweat glands are important in body temperature regulation. A human has from two to three million eccrine sweat glands covering almost all the body surface. They are particularly numerous on the palms of the hands and soles of the feet. Each sweat gland is a simple tubular gland consisting of a secretory coil deep in the dermis, and a duct which conveys the secreted sweat to the surface. Eccrine glands secrete water and electrolytes, lactate, urea and ammonia. The secretory coil produces isotonic sweat, but sodium chloride is reabsorbed in the duct so that sweat reaching the surface is hypotonic. Patients suffering from cystic fibrosis (mucoviscidosis) have defective resorption of sodium chloride and rapidly become salt depleted in a hot environment. Eccrine sweat glands are innervated by the sympathetic nervous sytem, but the neurotransmitter is acetylcholine.

Apocrine sweat glands

Apocrine sweat glands are found principally in the axillae and anogenital region. Specialized apocrine glands include the ceruminous glands of the external auditory meatus and the secretory milk glands of the breast. Apocrine glands, like eccrine glands, are composed of a secretory coil and a duct. The apocrine duct, however, opens into a hair follicle, and not directly onto the surface of the skin. Apocrine glands produce an oily secretion containing protein, carbohydrate, ammonia and lipid. These glands become active at puberty, and secretion is controlled by adrenergic nerve fibres. Pungent axillary body odour (axillary bromhidrosis) is the result of the action of bacteria on apocrine secretions. People with a good standard of hygiene have armpits whose bacterial flora is composed mainly of cocci, whereas Corynebacteria are the principal organisms in the bromhidrotic. In some animals apocrine secretions are important sexual attractants, but the average human armpit provides a different type of overwhelming olfactory experience.

Hair and sebaceous glands

Hairs grow out of tubular invaginations of the epidermis known as follicles, and a hair follicle and its associated sebaceous glands are referred to as a pilosebaceous unit. There are three types of hair. Lanugo hair is present *in utero* and shed by the eighth month of fetal life. Vellus hair is the fine downy hair which covers most of the body except those areas occupied by terminal hair. Terminal hair is the thick pigmented hair of the scalp, beard, eyebrows, eyelashes, axillae and pubic area. In some areas, such as the beard, axillae and pubic region, the development of terminal hair is under hormonal control—the hairs in these areas are vellus until the onset of puberty. On the scalp, the reverse occurs in male pattern balding—terminal hair becomes vellus hair. In men, terminal hair on the body usually increases in amount as middle age strikes, and hairy ears are a puzzling accompaniment of advancing years. One struggles to think of any possible biological advantage that hairy ears might confer.

Hair follicles extend into the dermis at an angle (Fig. 1.2). A small bundle of smooth muscle fibres, the arrector pili muscle, extends from just beneath the epidermis and is attached to the side of the follicle at an angle. Arrector pili muscles are supplied by adrenergic nerves, and are responsible for the erection of hairs during cold or emotional stress ('goose flesh'; horripilation). The sebaceous gland is attached to the follicle just above the point of attachment of the arrector pili. At the lower end of the follicle is the hair bulb, part of which, the hair matrix, is a zone of rapidly dividing cells which is responsible for the formation of the hair shaft. Hair pigment is produced by melanocytes in the hair bulb. Cells produced in the hair bulb become densely packed, elongated and arranged parallel to the long axis of the hair

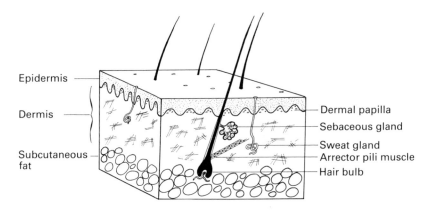

Epidermis

Dermis

Subcutaneous fat

Dermal papilla
Sebaceous gland
Sweat gland
Arrector pili muscle
Hair bulb

Fig. 1.2. The structure of the skin

shaft. They gradually become keratinized as they ascend in the hair follicle. The main part of each hair fibre is the cortex, which is composed of keratinized spindle-shaped cells (Fig. 1.3). Terminal hairs have a central core known as the medulla, consisting of specialized cells which contain air spaces. Covering the cortex is the cuticle, a thin layer of cells which overlap like the tiles on a roof, with the free margins of the cells pointing towards the tip of the hair. The cross-sectional shape of hair varies with body site and with race. Negroid hair is distinctly oval in cross-section, and pubic, beard and eyelash hairs are oval in all racial types.

The growth of each hair is cyclical—periods of active growth alternate with resting phases. After each period of active growth (anagen) there is a short resting phase (telogen), following which the follicle reactivates, a new hair is produced, and the old hair is shed. The duration of these cyclical phases depends on the age of the individual and the location of the follicle on the body. The duration of anagen in a scalp follicle is genetically

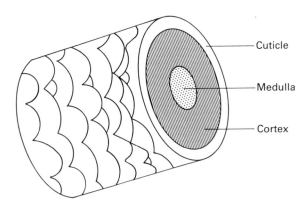

Cuticle

Medulla

Cortex

Fig. 1.3. The structure of hair.

determined, and ranges from 2 to >5 years. This is why some women can grow tresses down to the ankles, whereas most have a much shorter maximum length. Scalp hair telogen lasts from 3 to 4 months. The daily growth rate of scalp hair is approximately 0.35 mm. On the scalp the activity of each follicle is independent of that of its neighbour. This is fortunate, because if follicular activity was synchronized, as it is in some animals, we should be subject to periodic moults, which would add another dimension to life's rich tapestry. At any one time approximately 85% of scalp hairs are in anagen, and 15% in telogen. The average number of hairs shed daily is 100. In regions other than the scalp anagen is relatively short—this is also fortunate, for if it was not so, we should all be kept busy clipping eyebrows, eyelashes and nether regions.

It is a myth that shaving increases the rate of growth of hair and that it encourages 'thicker' hair. Nor does hair continue growing after death—shrinkage of soft tissues around the hair produces this illusion.

Human hair colour is produced by two types of melanin—eumelanins in black and brown hair, and phaeomelanins in auburn and blond hair.

Greying of hair with age is the result of a gradual decrease in tyrosinase activity in the melanocytes of the hair bulb. The age of onset of greying is principally genetically determined, but other factors may be involved such as autoimmunity—premature greying of the hair is a recognized association of pernicious anaemia. The phenomenon of 'going white overnight', usually associated with a severe fright, is physically impossible. It would, however, be feasible to 'go white' over a period of a few days by selective loss of pigmented hairs.

Sebaceous glands

Sebaceous glands are found everywhere on the skin apart from the palms of the hands and the soles and dorsa of the feet. They are particularly numerous and prominent on the head and neck, the front of the chest and back. Sebaceous glands are part of the pilosebaceous unit, and their lipid-rich secretion (sebum) flows through a duct into the hair follicle. Modified sebaceous glands which open directly on the surface are found on the eyelids, lips, nipples, glans penis and prepuce, and the buccal mucosa (Fordyce spots). They are holocrine glands—sebum is produced by disintegration of glandular cells rather than an active secretory process.

Sebaceous glands are prominent at birth, under the influence of maternal hormones, but atrophy soon after, and do not enlarge again until puberty. Enlargement of the glands and sebum production at puberty are stimulated by androgens. Growth hormone and thyroid hormones also affect sebum production.

Nails

A nail is a transparent plate of keratin derived from an invagination of epidermis on the dorsum of the terminal phalanx of a digit (Fig. 1.4). The nail plate is the product of cell division in the nail matrix, which lies deep to

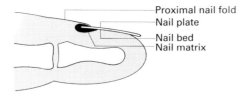

Proximal nail fold
Nail plate
Nail bed
Nail matrix

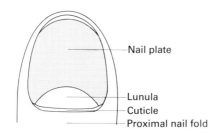

Nail plate

Lunula
Cuticle
Proximal nail fold

Fig. 1.4. The nail.

the proximal nail fold, but is partly visible as the pale 'half moon' (lunula) at the base of the nail. The part of the digit upon which the nail rests is known as the nail bed, and is thought not to contribute significantly to the formation of the nail plate. However, the nail plate firmly adheres to the nail bed. The cuticle is an extension of the horny layer of the proximal nail fold onto the nail plate. It is there to form a seal between the nail plate and proximal nail fold, preventing penetration of extraneous material, including bacteria, under the nail fold. A popular pastime amongst some ladies is the destruction of the cuticle by manicure implements or lytic chemicals, thus rendering them more susceptible to chronic paronychia (see Chapter 4).

Nail growth is continuous throughout life, but is more rapid in youth than in old age. The average rate of growth of finger nails is approximatley 1 mm per week, and the time taken for a finger nail to grow from matrix to free edge is about 6 months. Nails on the dominant hand grow slightly more rapidly than those on the other hand. Toe nails grow at about one-third the rate of finger nails, and take 18 months to grow from matrix to free edge.

Many factors can affect nail growth rate. The growth rate is increased in psoriasis, and may be speeded up in the presence of inflammatory change around the nail. A severe systemic upset can produce a sudden slowing of nail growth, and growth may be considerably slowed in a hand immobilized in plaster.

The dermis

The dermis is a layer of connective tissue lying beneath the epidermis and forming the bulk of the skin. The dermis and epidermis interdigitate via downward epidermal projections (rete ridges), and upward dermal projections (dermal papillae) (see Fig. 1.2). The main structural feature of the dermis is a network of interlacing fibres, mostly collagen, but with some elastin. These fibres give the dermis great strength and elasticity. The collagen and elastin fibres, which are protein, are embedded in a ground substance of mucopolysaccharides (glycosaminoglycans).

Fibroblasts, mast cells and macrophages constitute the main cellular elements of the dermis. Fibroblasts are responsible for the synthesis of the connective tissue matrix of the dermis, and are usually found in close proximity to collagen and elastin fibres. Mast cells are specialized secretory cells present throughout the dermis, but more numerous around blood vessels and appendages. The cytoplasm of mast cells contains granules whose contents include mediators such as histamine, prostaglandins, leukotrienes and eosinophil and neutrophil chemotactic factors. Mast cell degranulation occurs in immediate hypersensitivity reactions. Macrophages are phagocytic cells which originate in the bone marrow, and they act as scavengers of cell debris and extracellular material.

The dermis is also richly supplied with blood vessels, lymphatics, nerves, and sensory receptors.

Beneath the dermis a layer of subcutaneous fat separates the skin from underlying fascia and muscle.

Dermatoglyphics

Fingerprints, the characteristic elevated ridge patterns on the finger tips of humans, are unique to each individual. The fingers and toes, the palms of the hands and soles of the feet, are covered with a system of ridges which form certain patterns. The term dermatoglyphics is applied to both the configurations of the ridges, and also the study of fingerprints. If you look closely at the palms of your hands you will see these tiny ridges, which are quite separate from the skin creases. On the tips of the fingers there are three basic patterns—arches, loops and whorls (Fig. 1.5). The loops are subdivided into ulnar or radial, depending on whether the loop is open to the ulnar or radial side of the hand. A triangular intersection of these ridges is known as a triradius, and these triradii are not only present on fingertips, but also at the base of each finger, and usually on the proximal part of the palm.

(a)   (b)   (c)

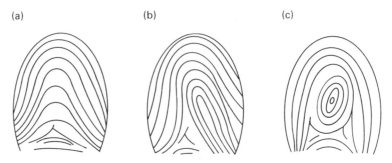

Fig. 1.5. Dermatoglyphics: (a) arch; (b) loop; (c) whorl.

Not only are the ridge patterns of fingerprints useful for the identification and conviction of those who covet their neighbours' goods, but characteristic dermatoglyphic abnormalities frequently accompany many chromosomal aberrations.

Functions of the skin

Skin is like wax paper that holds everything in without dripping.

(Art Linkletter,
A Child's Garden of Misinformation, 1965)

It is obvious from the complex structure of the skin that it is not there simply to hold all the other bits together. It is structured to prevent loss of essential body fluids, to protect the body against the entry of toxic environmental chemicals, to protect against damage from UV radiation, to regulate body temperature, and even to contribute to the body's supply of vitamin D.

In the absence of a stratum corneum we would all lose significant amounts of water to the environment, and rapidly become dehydrated. The stratum corneum with its overlapping cells and intercellular lipid, makes diffusion of water into the environment very difficult. If the stratum corneum is removed by stripping with tape, water loss to the environment increases 10-fold or more. Even with an intact stratum corneum we lose about 500 ml of water daily, mainly by diffusion through the skin.

The stratum corneum is also quite an effective barrier to external agents penetrating the skin. However, this barrier capacity is considerably reduced if the stratum corneum is hydrated, or its lipid content reduced by the use of lipid solvents. Hydration of the stratum corneum to reduce its barrier effect may be employed in the treatment of skin disease—the penetration of topical steroids can be increased by using an ointment base, a urea-containing base, or polythene occlusion, all of which hydrate the stratum corneum.

The protective effect of melanin in the skin against UV damage has already been mentioned.

The skin is a vital part of the body's temperature regulation system. The body core temperature is regulated by a temperature sensitive area in the hypothalamus, and this is influenced by the temperature of the blood perfusing it. The response to cold in the skin is vasoconstriction and a marked reduction in skin blood flow, decreasing transfer of heat to the body surface. The response to heat is vasodilatation, an increased skin blood flow, and loss of heat to the environment. Perspiration helps to cool the body by evaporation of the sweat. These thermoregulatory functions of the skin are impaired in certain skin diseases—for example patients suffering from exfoliative dermatitis radiate heat to their environment because their skin blood flow is enormously increased and they are unable to control this by vasoconstriction. In a cold environment their central core temperature would gradually drop and they would die of hypothermia.

The skin is also a huge sensory receptor, perceiving heat, cold, pain, temperature, light touch and pressure, and even tickle. As you are probably still pondering the biological advantages conferred by hairy ears, try switching your thoughts to the benefits of tickly armpits.

Vitamin D (cholecalciferol) is produced in the skin by the action of UV light on dehydrocholesterol. In those whose diets are deficient in vitamin D this extra source of the vitamin can be important.

So you can see that your skin is really doing quite a reasonable job. Apart from looking quite pleasant, it is saving you from becoming a cold, UV-damaged, brittle-boned, dessicated prune.

Chapter 2
Approach to the Diagnosis of Dermatological Disease

Baglivi has said, 'The patient is the doctor's best textbook'. That 'textbook' however has to be introduced to the student and those who effect the introductions are not always wise.

(Dannie Abse, in *Doctors and Patients*)

The dermatologist's art is giving a disease a long Greek name . . . and then a topical steroid.

We presume that, in picking up this little book and opening its pages, you are expressing some interest in learning about diseases of the skin. For most, it is likely that this interest has only arisen out of necessity, at least initially, and is expected to be a phase that will pass with time. It may, for example, have been forced upon you by your medical school office or you may, perhaps, have just seen a patient who has presented to you with a rash or a lump which you cannot deal with. We sincerely hope, however, that the interest which has led you to this volume will not disappear as soon as the dermatology term is over, or as soon as the patient has gone away. Dermatology is a fascinating branch of medicine which provides a stimulating range of diagnostic and therapeutic challenges. Dermatology is essentially a clinical specialty and it is important for any aspiring clinician to realize that, in order to be able to prescribe treatment and/or offer any useful prognostic information about a patient's problem, he or she must first make a diagnosis. This chapter is about that process in relation to dermatological disorders.

Value of a diagnosis

There is a great deal of truth in the comment attributed to Baglivi which forms part of Dannie Abse's quote at the head of this chapter. The facts on which a clinician makes his or her diagnosis must always come first and foremost from the patient and there is therefore no substitute for talking to and examining patients. This is especially true of skin disease.

There is also some truth in the second quote. It is one which we meet regularly in light-hearted conversation with our colleagues, when it is usually being used in a mildly derogatory way. However, there is actually nothing in the quote to be ashamed of. It merely emphasizes the importance that dermatologists place on making a primary diagnosis and their belief that this is the first fundamental step towards helping their patient. So what then is a diagnosis and what is involved in the process of making one?

A diagnosis is a short statement about a disease state or condition that has several important functions:

1   It provides a practical label which will be recognized by other doctors.

2 It implies a commonality of some feature or features with other patients suffering from the same disease state or condition. This may be in the cause (where known), the histopathological features, the clinical features or in the responsiveness to some form of treatment.

3 It offers a prognosis and information about the patient's chance of passing the disease on to others by contagion or heredity.

4 Finally, a diagnosis may provide access to treatment modalities.

Importance of experience

However, it is not enough to examine patients in a vacuum. In order to reach a diagnosis, the doctor must use all the information at his disposal and, although some teachers imply that it is possible to reach diagnoses from first principles, most of us accept that we make the majority of our diagnoses from experience. This experience has to be achieved by a combination of exposure and information provided from outside. This usually comes from one's books, teachers and peers. Perhaps an illustration will help you to see what we mean.

Imagine that you are the first person to land on Mars and that you have found your way into a Martian supermarket. As you walk between the shelves you see hundreds of objects you have never seen in your life before. You have never seen pictures of Martian goods in a book and no one has told you what you might expect to find. At the end of the row a Martian supervisor asks you to name everything you have just seen. Obviously you cannot. You have to ask the Martian to tell you—and even then you will not remember them all immediately. However, you will remember some and you will be able to name them the second time round. If you were to stay on Mars, you would gradually become familiar with all the objects on sale, although you would probably have to ask the name of some several times from your new-found friends or the Martian supervisor, or look them up in a catalogue.

This is, in essence, what we are all doing as we try to become better diagnosticians. The process begins with exposure to patients, but just taking a history and examining patients is not enough. The learning process must also involve some form of audit or feedback. It is here that the quality of the student's teacher or textbooks is so important. If the teacher or textbook tell the student that an apple is a pear or that psoriasis is eczema or even that black is white, the student will continue to believe this until something or someone else teaches him otherwise. It is through this process that you will begin to be familiar with the diagnostic labels in use in dermatology.

Please now re-read Dannie Abse's full quote at the head of this chapter.

Dermatological diagnosis

The aspiring dermatologist must begin by becoming familiar with the diagnostic labels used in the description and classification of skin disease. This can seem daunting at first glance, but it is important to remember that currently accepted diagnostic entities in clinical medicine are bound by convention. Dermatology is no different from other specialties, except perhaps in the degree to which subtle clinical variations are afforded their own separate name. The names given to disease states have emerged by a general concensus from attempts at classifying and categorizing diseases which have been going on for many hundreds of years. Although many people seem to find it distressing that diagnostic terms in use often bear no real relationship to modern understanding of the disease, this is not of itself important. For example, we all understand what is meant by the word 'apple', even though most of us have no idea why it is used to describe that particular fruit. A good dermatological example of this is psoriasis (see Chapter 8). Literally, 'psoriasis' simply means the 'itchy condition', but the term has come to represent a very well-defined clinicopathological entity. When one doctor says 'psoriasis' to another, both will understand what is meant (or at least they ought to!).

Therefore, as in any other branch of medicine, the diagnostic terminology currently in use in dermatology will have to be learned. This is not as hard as it may at first seem. In the same way as the visitor to Mars will become familiar with Martian goods, so the aspiring dermatologist will rapidly become acquainted with the commoner skin diseases such as eczema, psoriasis or warts. In time, he or she will also begin to recognize rarer disorders and also less 'classical' variants of the commoner ones. However, as mentioned above, this is a dynamic process which involves seeing, reading, asking and learning— always with the eyes, ears and mind open!

In trying to learn about dermatological disease, therefore, we believe that you should certainly try to see as many patients as possible but that you should also read around the disorders you meet, discuss them with your colleagues and never be afraid to ask your teachers to explain the 'why's' the 'what's' and the 'wherefore's'.

Steps to making a dermatological diagnosis

There is nothing difficult in principle about dermatological diagnosis. As with any other specialty, the process of identifying skin diseases consists of taking a history, examining the patient and, where necessary, performing some investigations.

History-taking

Fundamental elements:
    Presenting complaint
    Past history
      General
      Skin disease
      Allergies
    Family history
      General
      Skin disease
    Occupation/hobbies
    Treatment
      Topical
      Systemic

The dermatological history contains most of the elements that you are used to taking in other wards or clinics, such as onset and duration, fluctuation, nature of symptoms, past history and so on. There are some differences, however, which are largely in the emphasis placed on certain aspects.

Patients with skin disease will talk about symptoms, such as itching, which you may not have met before. You will have to learn to assess and quantify these. For example, a severe itch will keep patients awake or stop them from concentrating at work. However, you will soon get used to this. Do be careful, too, about the terms the patients use themselves to describe their skin problems. In our part of the country it is common to find weals being called 'blisters' and it is easy to be misled. The visible evidence is there for all to see: the patient, his/her spouse, father, mother, grandfather, the local vet, the greengrocer, the local policeman and the next-door neighbour can all see the problem and express their opinion. Always ask the patient to describe precisely what he or she means by a specific term.

It is also important when taking a good dermatological history to pay special attention to certain aspects:

1 *Past history* This obviously includes general problems, such as diabetes and TB, but should also include past skin problems and any significant allergies.

2 *Family history* This is because some disorders, such as scabies are infectious, and because others, such as eczema and psoriasis have strong genetic backgrounds.

3 *Occupation and hobbies* The skin is frequently affected by materials in the workplace and in the home or potting shed.

4 *Systemic and topical therapy* Not only may systemic medication affect the skin but many patients apply multiple creams and ointments to their skin. These may be medicinal and patients nearly always forget their names. Additionally many people literally plaster themselves with creams, lotions and salves as part of a 'cosmetic' regime.

Examination

Fundamental elements:

Site and/or distribution

Characteristics of individual lesion(s)

Special techniques

Your next step is to examine the patient. Wise counsels maintain that you should always examine the patient from head to foot. In reality this can be hard on both patient and doctor, especially if the presenting complaint is a solitary wart on the thumb! However, as a general rule and especially when dealing with inflammatory dermatoses and other conditions where there are several lesions rather than a solitary lump, it is very important to have an overall look at the sites involved. You may also turn up useful, unexpected findings, like melanomas and other skin cancers.

Examination should involve a careful inspection and palpation of the lesion(s) or rash. It may be helpful to use a magnifying hand lens. The examination of the skin should take note of two fundamental features:

1   *The site(s) and/or distribution of the lesion(s)* This can be very helpful. For example, psoriasis has a predilection for the knees, elbows, scalp and the base of the spine; eczema favours the flexures in children; acne occurs predominantly on the face and upper trunk; basal cell carcinomas are more common on the head and neck.

2   *The characteristics of the individual lesion* This is an area in which you will certainly need to do some preliminary reading before approaching the patient. You need to have some familiarity with the terms used to describe dermatological conditions.

Unfortunately, names and terms often appear to get in the way of learning in dermatology more than in some other specialties. Indeed this seems to be an important reason for many clinicians claiming that dermatology is a mysterious mixture of mumbo-jumbo and strange potions which is virtually impossible to penetrate. There is really no need for this attitude. The terms in use have developed for entirely valid reasons. They provide us with a degree of precision and a framework for diagnosis and decision-making.

The most important ones are listed in Table 2.1.

It is important that you try to become familiar with these terms and try to apply them correctly. This will help to provide the building-blocks with which you will then go on to make dermatological diagnoses. Each of these terms has a precise meaning and needs no further definition.

The individual lesions will, in the early days, be described in the terms listed below. However, in most inflammatory dermatoses it is not always quite as simple as this because you have to decide which lesion or lesions to select for this descriptive process. Skin diseases are dynamic. In any eruption some lesions will be very early, some very late and some at various evolutionary stages in between. Part of the value of the experience that comes with frequent

Table 2.1. Terms commonly used to describe skin changes

Macule	A flat, circumscribed area of skin discolouration
Papule	A circumscribed elevation of the skin <1 cm in diameter
Nodule	A circumscribed palpable lump, >1 cm in diameter
Plaque	A circumscribed, disc-shaped, elevated area of skin, >1 cm in diameter
Vesicle	A small visible collection of fluid (<1 cm in diameter)
Bulla	A large visible collection of fluid (>1 cm in diameter)
Pustule	A visible accumulation of pus
Ulcer	A loss of epidermis (often with loss of underlying dermis and subcutis as well)
Scale	Visible and palpable flakes due to aggregation and/or abnormalities of shed epidermal cells
Crust	Accumulated dried exudate, e.g. serum
Weal	A circumscribed, elevated area of cutaneous oedema
Excoriation	A secondary, superficial ulceration, which is due to scratching

examination of skin diseases is that you develop an ability to pick those lesions which give the most useful diagnostic information.

There are, in addition to simple inspection and palpation, some little tricks that can be used in certain situations to provide extra information. These will be dealt with later in the appropriate sections of the book, but it is worth mentioning some examples here: scraping the surface of psoriatic lesions will induce capillary point haemorrhage; the Nikolsky sign, where the skin shears off around the erosions of pemphigus and toxic epidermal necrolysis; diascopy (pressing on a lesion with a glass slide) is useful in diagnosing lupus vulgaris.

This diagnostic process will gradually become one which you perform increasingly easily and increasingly confidently as experience develops.

Investigation

Fundamental elements:
  Blood tests
  Swabs
  Wood's light
  Scrapes/clips
    Microscopy
    Mycological culture
  Skin biopsy
    Histopathology
    Electron microscopy
    Immunopathology
  Patch tests

Inevitably, the history and examination alone will not always provide all the information required for the best management of the patient. There are some skin disorders in which further investigation is nearly always necessary: either to confirm a diagnosis with important prognostic or therapeutic implications (e.g. blistering disorders), or to seek an underlying, associated systemic disorder (e.g. in generalized pruritus). These situations will generally be covered in the appropriate chapters later in the book. Sometimes, of course, clinical findings alone will not produce a satisfactory working diagnosis or further information will be required in order to provide optimal management for the patient. We should therefore discuss briefly at this point the most important techniques that are available to help achieve a diagnosis. Some of these, such as appropriate blood tests and swabs for bacteriology and virology, should be familiar from other branches of medicine and are fully covered in other introductory textbooks. Others, however, are more specific to dermatological investigation.

Wood's light

This is UV light with a special nickel oxide filter over the light source. It may be used to highlight three relatively common features of cutaneous disease:

1   Certain fungi causing scalp ringworm produce green fluorescence. This is useful in the initial diagnosis and may be helpful in assessing the efficacy of therapy.

2 The organism responsible for erythrasma fluoresces coral-pink under Wood's light.

3 Some pigmentary disorders are much more clearly visible if viewed under UV light. Particularly important are the pale patches seen in tuberous sclerosis and café-au-lait marks in neurofibromatosis.

Wood's light can also be used to induce fluorescence in the urine in porphyrias.

Scrapings/clippings

It is often useful to take some superficial material from the skin, hair or nails for direct examination under the microscope or for culture, particularly in a suspected fungal infection, molluscum contagiosum or in a search for the scabies mite (see Chapters 3, 4, 5). The best tool for taking skin scrapings is the 'banana' scalpel. The area under investigation is scraped lightly with the scalpel, which will bring off scales from the surface. It may be worth wiping off any ointment first with some alcohol. The scales thus obtained are placed on a microscope slide and covered with a solution of 10% potassium hydroxide (KOH) and a cover slip. They can be examined directly within a few minutes (to allow dissolution of some of the epidermal cell membranes). It may be helpful to add one or two drops of ink if the organism being sought is *Pityrosporum* (the cause of pityriasis versicolor). Nail clippings can also be treated in this manner but need much stronger solutions of KOH, or a longer period of time to dissolve before examination. Similarly, microscopy of hair may provide useful information about possible fungal infections but it may also reveal structural abnormalities of the hair shaft in certain genetic disorders, and can be used in the diagnosis of some conditions where there is excessive hair loss (see Chapter 13).

Scrape/smear preparations are also used by some dermatologists for the purpose of cytodiagnosis (Tzanck preparation). The main applications are suspected viral blisters and suspected pemphigus. The advantage of the technique is that suitably stained material can be examined directly in the clinic, but very few dermatologists would rely on this alone and in most circumstances would send swabs and/or a biopsy as well.

Skin biopsy

Skin biopsies are a fundamental part of the diagnostic process in many skin disorders. In some conditions it is critical to have confirmation of a clinical diagnosis before embarking on treatment. Good examples of this are skin cancers, bullous disorders and infections such as tuberculosis and leprosy. In others it is necessary to take a biopsy because clinical information alone has not provided all the answers.

There are two methods commonly used to obtain a skin sample for laboratory examination: the incisional/excision biopsy and the punch biopsy. The first of these techniques is illustrated in Fig. 2.1, and the equipment required is shown in Fig. 2.2. The first step is normally to administer a local

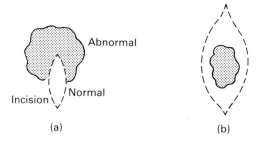

Fig. 2.1 The technique for incisional/excisional biopsy.

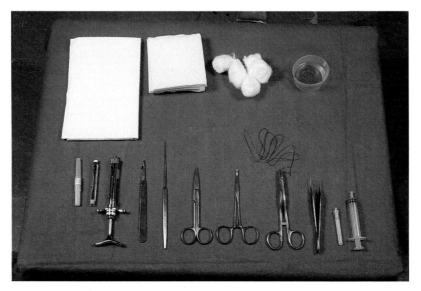

Fig. 2.2 The equipment for an incisional/excisional biopsy: sterile towel; gauze squares; cotton wool balls; galley pot containing antiseptic; needle; cartridge of lignocaine and dental syringe; scalpel; skin hook; scissors; small artery forceps; needle holder and suture; fine, toothed forceps; needle and syringe (alternative to dental syringe).

anaesthetic. This is usually lignocaine in a 1% solution. The addition of adrenaline is a concentration of 1 : 10 000 is a useful aid in reducing bleeding, but should NOT be used on extremities.

For an *incisional*, diagnostic biopsy two cuts are made to form an ellipse. It is important to ensure that the specimen is taken across the edge of the lesion being biopsied, retaining a margin of normal perilesional skin (Fig. 2.1(a)). For complete *excision*, the ellipse is widened to take in the whole lesion (Fig. 2.1 (b)). It is important to ensure that the excision edge is cut vertically and does not tend to slant in towards the tumour, as this can result in inadequate deeper excision (Fig. 2.3). The edges of the defect left by either incisional or excisional

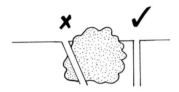

Fig. 2.3. Excisional biopsy: the correct (tick) and incorrect (cross) excision edge.

biopsy can be brought neatly together with sutures. The choice of suture material is not critical, but if the cosmetic result is important, it should be as fine as possible and a man-made monofilament suture (e.g. prolene) is probably the most satisfactory.

The second technique—punch biopsy (Fig. 2.4(a)–(c))—is much quicker. After anaesthetizing the skin, a hollow, circular knife blade (or 'punch') is pressed firmly into the lesion being biopsied and turned gently. This releases a small plug, which is then lifted gently out and cut free with scissors or a scalpel. Haemostasis can be achieved with a silver nitrate stick and the defect is usually small enough to be left to heal by secondary intention, although it is also possible to close the area with a suture.

The specimens thus obtained may be sent for conventional histopathology, in which case they will normally be fixed in formalsaline. However, in some instances, there will be a need for other specialized examinations instead of, or in addition to, conventional examination. For immunological examination the skin needs to be snap frozen and for electron microscopy it is best fixed in glutaraldehyde. It is important to check these details with the laboratory before you start.

Patch tests

If a contact allergic dermatitis is suspected, it is necessary to perform a patch test. This is a process in which a possible allergen is placed in contact with the skin (usually of the back) for 48 h to see if there is a reaction. The allergens are generally diluted in suitable vehicles and are applied on inert tapes or in small discs (Fig. 2.5). A positive reaction confirms a delayed hypersensitivity (Type IV) to the offending substance.

These techniques can be extended to include testing for photo-allergy.

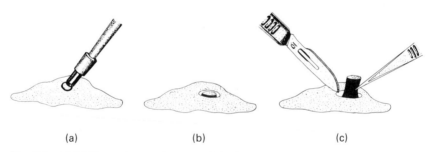

(a)   (b)   (c)

Fig. 2.4. (a)-(c) The technique for a punch biopsy.

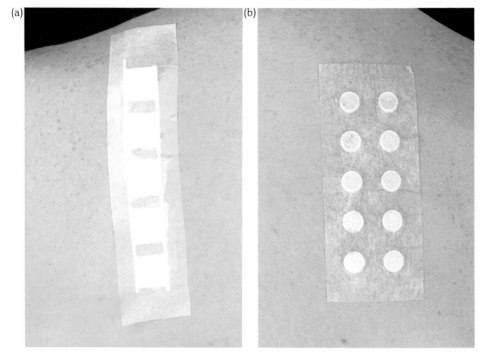

Fig. 2.5. Patch testing: (a) aluminium strip under tape; (b) metal cups under tape.

Conclusion

You are now armed with enough information to start examining patients with skin disease. What you should do now is to attend some dermatology clinics and start trying to put these principles into practice. When seeing patients, try to retain a mental picture of them and their skin lesions. Ask the dermatologist in charge what the diagnosis is in each instance and then make sure that you read a little about each entity when the clinic is over.

The remaining chapters of this book are designed to help to provide some of the information you will require to fill in the background and, hopefully, to be able eventually to make specific diagnoses.

Chapter 3
Bacterial and Viral Infections

A mighty creature is the germ,
Though smaller than the pachyderm.
His customary dwelling place
Is deep within the human race.
His childish pride he often pleases
By giving people strange diseases.
Do you, my poppet, feel infirm?
You probably contain a germ.
          (Ogden Nash, The Germ)

Bacterial infections

Streptococcal infection

Cellulitis

Cellulitis is an infection of the skin and subcutaneous tissues by *Streptococcus pyogenes*. Superficial streptococcal infection of the skin is often called 'erysipelas', but a separate term seems unnecessary, as it is often impossible to judge the depth of tissue involved.

The legs are a common site for cellulitis, but other parts of the body, including the face, may be affected. The organisms probably gain entry into the skin via minor abrasions. A frequent predisposing factor is lower limb oedema, and cellulitis is a common condition in the elderly, who often suffer from leg oedema. Stasis ulcers provide a portal of entry for the organisms in some cases. The affected area becomes erythematous, hot, and swollen (Fig. 3.1), and occasionally blister formation and areas of skin necrosis occur. The patient is pyrexial and feels unwell. Rigors may occur, and, in the elderly, a toxic confusional state.

Strict bed rest is important in treatment. Cellulitis should be treated with parenteral penicillin. If extensive areas of tissue necrosis occur, surgical debridement may be necessary.

Some patients have recurrent episodes of cellulitis, each episode damaging lymphatics and leading to further oedema. These cases should be treated with prophylactic oral penicillin V or erythromycin, to prevent further cellulitic episodes.

Staphylococcal infection

Folliculitis

Infection of the superficial part of a hair follicle with *Staph. aureus* produces a small pustule on an erythematous base, centred on the follicle. Folliculitis is a common problem in eczema patients treated with ointment-based topical steroid preparations.

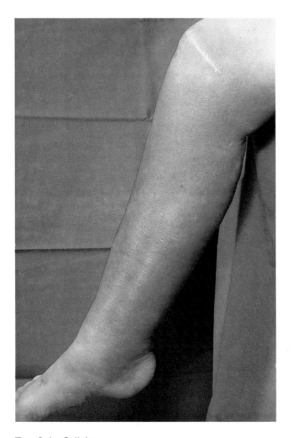

Fig. 3.1. Cellulitis.

Mild folliculitis can be treated with a topical antibacterial agent, but if extensive a systemic antibiotic may be required.

Furunculosis ('boils')

A boil is the result of deep infection of a hair follicle by *Staph. aureus*. A painful inflammatory nodule develops at the site of infection, and over a period of a few days becomes fluctuant and 'points' as a central pustule. Once the central necrotic core has been discharged, the lesion gradually resolves. In some patients boils are a recurrent problem, but this is rarely associated with a significant underlying disorder. Usually, such individuals are carriers of staphylococci in the nose, or on the perineum, and the organisms are carried on the digits to various parts of the body.

Patients suffering from recurrent boils should have swabs taken from the nose for culture, and if found to be carrying staphylococci should be treated with a topical antibacterial such as Naseptin cream or Bactroban Nasal. They may also be helped by the use of Ster-Zac Bath Concentrate (2% triclosan) when bathing, and a prolonged course of cloxacillin or flucloxacillin.

Carbuncle

A carbuncle is a deep infection of a group of adjacent hair follicles with *Staph. aureus*. A frequent site for a carbuncle is the nape of the neck. Initially the lesion is a dome-shaped area of tender erythema, but after a few days suppuration begins, and pus is discharged from multiple follicular orifices. Carbuncles are usually encountered in middle-aged and elderly men, and are frequently associated with diabetes or severe debility. Cloxacillin or flucloxacillin should be given for treatment, and the abscesses drained.

Impetigo

This is a superficial bacterial infection of the skin caused by *Staph. aureus*, or a combination of this organism and haemolytic streptoccocci. Lesions may occur anywhere on the body, but the head and neck area is frequently affected. The initial lesion is a small pustule which rapidly increases in size, and soon ruptures to leave a raw, exuding surface. The exudate dries to form a golden yellow crust, and the stratum corneum peels back at the margins of the affected area to give a typical appearance (Fig. 3.2). Impetigo may occur as a secondary phenomenon in atopic eczema, scabies and head louse infestation.

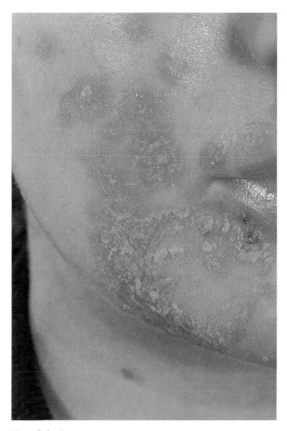

Fig. 3.2. Impetigo.

Except in the most localized cases, impetigo should be treated with a systemic antibiotic such as cloxacillin, flucloxacillin or erythromycin. Many staphylococci are penicillinase-producers and are therefore resistant to penicillin. A useful topical antibacterial agent to use on localized cases, or as an adjunct to systemic therapy, is mupirocin 2% (Bactroban ointment).

Staphylococcal scalded skin syndrome

This condition occurs as a result of infection with certain staphylococcal phage types which produce a toxin which splits the epidermis at the level of the granular layer. The superficial epidermis peels off in sheets, and the appearance resembles severe scalding. Infants and young children are those usually affected, but fortunately the condition is uncommon. It responds well to treatment with cloxacillin or flucloxacillin.

Erysipeloid

This is an infection with the organism *Erysipelothrix rhusiopathiae,* and may afflict those handling uncooked meat, poultry, fish and shellfish. It is therefore seen in butchers, slaughterhouse workers, fishermen and fishmongers. The organism enters the skin via an abrasion, and produces a well-defined purplish red area which spreads gradually. There is no constitutional upset. It responds to treatment with penicillin.

Erythrasma

This is a condition produced by a Gram-positive bacillus, *Corynebacterium minutissimum.* Erythrasma typically occurs in intertriginous areas—axillae, groins and submammary regions, but the commonest site colonized by this organism is the toe web-spaces. In the web-spaces it produces a macerated scaling appearance identical to that produced by fungal infection. In the other sites of predilection the clinical appearance is of marginated brown areas with a fine, branny surface scale (Fig. 3.3). It is usually asymptomatic. *C. minutissimum* produces a porphyrin which fluoresces a striking coral-pink under Wood's light.

Erythrasma may be treated with topical imidazoles (clotrimazole, miconazole, econazole), topical fusidic acid (Fucidin), or a 2-week course of oral erythromycin.

Mycobacterial infection

Cutaneous tuberculosis

Cutaneous tuberculosis is now becoming rare in the indigenous population of Great Britain but it is occasionally encountered in the immigrant population, particularly those from the Indian subcontinent.

Lupus vulgaris

This is a postprimary cutaneous infection with *Mycobacterium tuberculosis.* In some cases the bacilli reach the skin by haematogenous spread from another

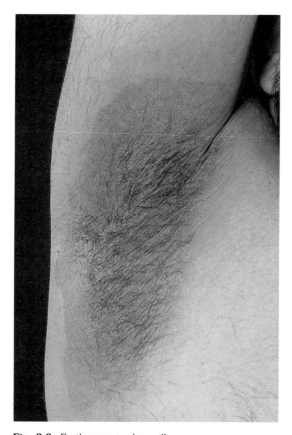

Fig. 3.3. Erythrasma in the axilla.

site, in others by lymphatic extension from tuberculous cervical adenitis, but in many the origin of the infection cannot be determined.

The lesions of lupus vulgaris are found on the head and neck in over 90% of cases. The typical appearance is of a reddish brown, nodular plaque with a scaly surface (Fig. 3.4). When pressed with a glass slide (diascopy), the brown nodules are more easily seen, and are referred to as 'apple jelly nodules'—this is, I am sure, an apt comparison, provided one is cognizant with the appearance of apple jelly. The natural course of these lesions is gradual peripheral extension, and in many cases this is extremely slow. Active lupus vulgaris is a destructive process, and the cartilage of nose and ears may be severely damaged.

Histology shows tubercles composed of epithelioid cells and Langhans giant cells, usually without central caseation. Tubercle bacilli are present in very small numbers, and can rarely be demonstrated by staining. The Mantoux test is strongly positive. The patient should be investigated for an underlying focus of tuberculosis in other organs, but such a focus is only found in approximately 10% of cases.

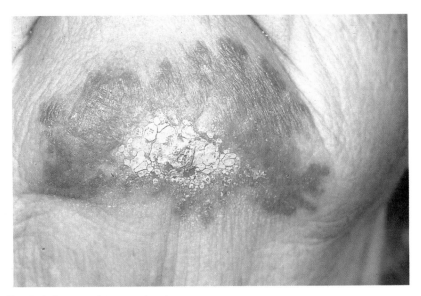

Fig. 3.4. Lupus vulgaris on the chin.

Treatment should be with standard antituberculous chemotherapy. In the absence of a focus in another organ, lupus vulgaris may be effectively treated with a combination of two drugs—for example rifampicin and isoniazid ('Rifinah'). (Don't forget the pyridoxine.)

There is a risk of the development of squamous cell carcinoma in the scar tissue of long-standing lupus vulgaris.

Warty tuberculosis

This is a chronic warty type of tuberculosis which occurs as a result of direct inoculation of tubercle bacilli into the skin of someone previously infected, and having a high degree of immunity. In the East it is the commonest variety of cutaneous tuberculosis, occurring predominantly on the buttocks and thighs, as a result of sitting on ground contaminated by infected sputum. It responds very well to standard antituberculous chemotherapy.

Tuberculids

This term is applied to a group of disorders which occur as an immunological response to tuberculosis elsewhere in the body. Included in this group are papulonecrotic tuberculid, lichen scrofulosorum and erythema induratum (Bazin's disease).

Leprosy (Hansen's disease)

If the possibility of leprosy enters into the discussion of differential diagnosis at the bedside, the eponymous title of this condition should always be used, because the fear of leprosy is still so ingrained, even in countries where it is not endemic. The Norwegian Armauer Hansen discovered the leprosy bacillus, *M.*

leprae, in 1873. Leprosy has a wide distribution throughout the world, with the majority of cases occurring in the tropics and subtropics. In Great Britain the disease is confined to immigrants, and those who have lived in endemic areas.

Leprosy is essentially a disease of peripheral nerves, but it also affects the skin, and sometimes other tissues such as the eyes, the mucosa of the upper respiratory tract, the bones and the testes. Although it is an infectious disease, the degree of infectivity is low. The incubation period is lengthy, probably several years, and it is likely that most patients acquire the infection in childhood. The disease is acquired as a result of close physical contact with an infected individual, the risk being much greater for contacts of lepromatous cases, but the portal of entry of the bacillus into the human body is unknown.

The clinical pattern of disease is determined by the host's cell-mediated immune response to the organism. When this is well-developed the pattern of disease is tuberculoid leprosy, in which skin and peripheral nerves are affected. Skin lesions are single, or few in number, and are well-defined. They are macules or plaques which are hypopigmented in dark skin. The lesions are anaesthetic, sweating is absent within the affected areas of skin, and hairs are reduced in number or absent. Thickened branches of cutaneous sensory nerves may be palpable in the region of the lesions, and large peripheral nerves may also be palpable. The lepromin test is strongly positive. Histology shows well-defined tuberculoid granulomas, and bacilli are not seen on modified Ziehl–Neelsen staining.

When the cell-mediated immune response to the bacilli is poor, the bacilli multiply unchecked, and the pattern of disease is that of lepromatous leprosy. The bacilli spread to involve not only the skin, but also the mucosa of the respiratory tract, the eyes, testes and bones. The skin lesions are multiple and nodular. The lepromin test is negative. Histology shows a diffuse granuloma throughout the dermis, and bacilli are present in large numbers.

In between these two extreme, 'polar' forms of leprosy is a spectrum of disease referred to as borderline leprosy, the clinical and histological features of which reflect different degrees of cell-mediated response to the bacilli. There is no absolute diagnostic test for leprosy—the diagnosis is based on clinical and histological features.

Tuberculoid leprosy is usually treated with a combination of dapsone and rifampicin; lepromatous leprosy with dapsone, rifampicin and clofazimine. The treatment of leprosy may be complicated by immunologically mediated 'reactional states', and should be supervised by someone experienced in leprosy management.

Atypical mycobacteria

The commonest of the skin lesions produced by atypical mycobacteria is the 'swimming-pool' or 'fish-tank' granuloma. This is often a solitary granulomatous nodule, caused by inoculation of *M. marinum* into the skin via an abrasion—sustained whilst swimming, or in tropical fish fanciers whilst cleaning out the aquarium. Occasionally, in addition to the initial lesion, there are multiple secondary lesions in a linear distribution along the lines of lymphatics.

Conventional antituberculous chemotherapy is often not very effective against *M. marinum*, but minocycline or cotrimoxazole have been found to be helpful in treatment.

Treponemal disease

Syphilis

Syphilis simulates every other disease. It is the only disease necessary to know. Know syphilis in all its manifestations and relations, and all other things clinical will be added to you.

(Sir William Osler)

Syphilis is a sexually transmitted disease caused by the spirochaete *Treponema pallidum*. There has been a gradual decline in the incidence of syphilis in the Western world during this century, and the late forms of syphilis are now extremely rare. The decline in the incidence of early syphilis has not been quite as dramatic, and in recent decades there has been an increased rate of infection in homosexual men.

Syphilis has an incubation period of 3–4 weeks at the end of which a primary sore (chancre) develops at the site of inoculation of the organism. Primary chancres occur most commonly on the penis and vulva, but other sites include the cervix, anal canal, nipples, lips and fingers. The chancre develops as a small papule which rapidly ulcerates. The ulcer is usually solitary, painless, and has an indurated base with an erythematous halo. *T. pallidum* can be demonstrated on dark field illumination of serum from the base of the ulcer. The chancre usually heals in 2–6 weeks. Serological tests for syphilis become positive in the later part of the primary stage.

Several weeks, sometimes several months, after the primary lesion has healed, the secondary stage appears. This is usually characterized by mild constitutional upset, generalized lymphadenopathy, a non-itchy rash, and lesions on the mucous membranes. Classically the skin lesions seen in secondary syphilis are copper-coloured papules scattered over the trunk and limbs, and characteristically affecting the palms and soles. However, the skin lesions may be psoriasiform, or resemble pityriasis rosea. In warm, moist areas, such as the perineum, the papules enlarge into pink or grey discs (condylomata lata) which contain large numbers of organisms and are highly infectious. Painless erosions (mucous patches) may develop in the mouth, and form circles or arcs (snail-track ulcers). These also contain large numbers of organisms and are highly infectious. A less common manifestation is a patchy alopecia (moth-eaten alopecia). All these features eventually disappear spontaneously.

In 30–40% of untreated cases a tertiary stage develops several years later. The skin lesions seen in tertiary syphilis are either granulomatous nodular lesions or gummata. A typical gumma is a punched-out ulcer with a slough in its base, likened to chamois leather.

Penicillin is the treatment of choice for syphilis. Treatment and contact tracing should be undertaken in a department of genitourinary medicine.

Viral infections

Warts

> Fasting spittle is good for warts.
> (Traditional English)

Warts are benign epidermal neoplasms caused by viruses of the human papilloma virus (HPV) group. There are a number of different strains of HPV which produce different clinical types of warts. Warts are also known as verrucae, although the term verruca in popular usage is usually reserved for the plantar wart.

Common warts

These are raised, cauliflower-like lesions which occur most frequently on the hands. They are extremely common in childhood and early adult life. They may be scattered, grouped or periungual in distribution. Common warts in children usually resolve spontaneously.

Common warts are usually treated with wart paints or cryotherapy. Preparations containing salicylic acid (e.g. Salactol—salicylic acid and lactic acid in collodion), glutaraldehyde (e.g. Glutarol) or formaldehyde (e.g. Veracur gel) are often quite effective, and a wart paint should certainly be used for at least 3 months before considering alternative treatment. Cryotherapy with liquid nitrogen can be used on warts resistant to treatment with wart paints. A simple applicator of cotton wool wrapped around the end of an orange stick is dipped in the nitrogen and applied to the wart until it and a narrow rim of surrounding skin are frozen. It is a painful procedure, and should not be inflicted on small children—most tiny tots will, in any case, have retreated under the desk at the sight of the nitrogen evaporating in its container. Multiple warts usually require more than one application, and the optimum interval between treatments is 3 weeks.

Plantar warts

Plantar warts may be solitary, scattered over the sole of the foot, or grouped together producing so-called mosaic warts (Fig. 3.5). The typical appearance of a plantar wart is of a small area of thickened skin which when pared away reveals several black dots produced by thrombosed capillaries. Plantar warts are frequently painful on walking. They must be distinguished from calluses and corns, which develop in areas of friction over bony prominences. Calluses are patches of uniformly thickened skin, and corns have a painful central plug of keratin which does not contain capillaries.

Wart paints are the mainstay of treatment for planter warts—cryotherapy is not as effective as it is on hand warts, but is often used in combination with wart paints. Occasionally, resistant warts may be removed by curettage, but they should never be excised as a permanent painful scar may be produced.

A question frequently asked is whether children with plantar warts should be barred from using public swimming-baths because of the risk of transmission of

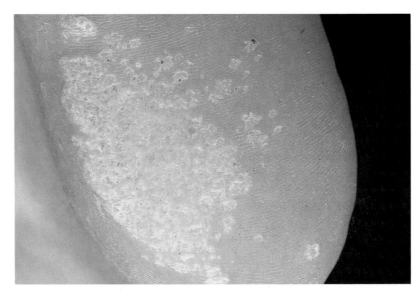

Fig. 3.5. Mosaic plantar warts.

the wart virus to others. Most dermatologists consider this is somewhat Draconian, and its enforcement would empty most public baths in the land.

Plane warts
These are tiny, flat-topped, flesh-coloured warts which usually occur on the dorsa of the hands and the face (Fig. 3.6). They often occur in lines due to inoculation of the virus into scratches and abrasions. Plane warts are extremely difficult to treat effectively, and attempts at treatment may do more harm than good. They will resolve spontaneously eventually, and are best left alone.

Genital warts (condylomata acuminata)
In recent years the importance of certain types of genital wart viruses in the aetiology of penile and cervical cancer has been recognized, and this has modified attitudes to what was previously considered a minor sexually transmitted inconvenience. It is now perhaps more appropriate that patients suffering from genital warts are seen and treated in a department of genitourinary medicine, so that coexisting sexually transmitted disease can be detected, and sexual contacts traced and examined.

Warts on the penis, vulva and perianal area are usually small cauliflower-like excrescences (Fig. 3.7), but occasionally proliferate into huge warty masses. They may be treated by the application of compound podophyllin paint (in concentrations of between 5% and 25%) at weekly intervals. Podophyllin is an irritant, and the paint should not be allowed to stay on the skin longer than 6 h before being washed off. It is also toxic if absorbed, and should not be used in large quantities, or in the treatment of pregnant women with genital warts.

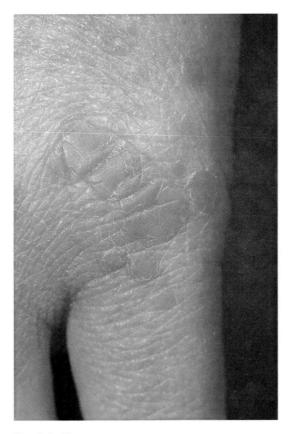

Fig. 3.6. Plane warts.

Genital warts may also be treated by cryotherapy, and if they are very florid are best dealt with by cautery under anaesthetic.

Molluscum contagiosum

The lesions of molluscum contagiosum are caused by a pox virus. They are typically pearly pink papules with a central umbilication filled with a horny plug (Fig. 3.8). The lesions may occur anywhere on the body, but are most commonly encountered on the head and neck area and the trunk. They are frequently grouped, and may be surrounded by a mild eczematous reaction. They may be very extensive in children with atopic eczema.

There is no antiviral agent which has any effect on the virus causing these lesions, but their natural history is for eventual spontaneous resolution. In infants and young children they are best left to resolve spontaneously, but if parents are anxious that something more positive be done they can be advised to gently squeeze each lesion between the thumb nails to express the central plug—this will often speed their resolution. In older children and adults molluscum contagiosum can be treated by cryotherapy, or by carefully pricking the centre of each lesion with phenol on the end of a cocktail stick.

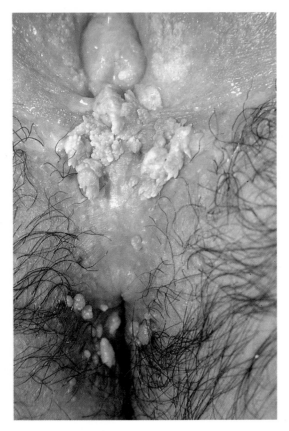

Fig. 3.7. Genital warts.

Orf

Orf is a viral disease of sheep which produces multiple lesions around the mouth. The virus can be transmitted to humans, and those usually affected are women who bottle-feed lambs, and butchers and slaughterhouse workers who handle the carcasses of sheep. The typical clinical picture is of a solitary inflammatory papule which rapidly develops into a domed nodule of granulation tissue—usually on a finger (Fig. 3.9), but occasionally the lesion is on the face, and rarely there are multiple lesions. The diagnosis can be confirmed by electron microscopy of smears from the granulation tissue. Orf lesions resolve spontaneously in 6–8 weeks. The antiviral agent idoxuridine is said to have some activity against the orf virus, and may be used topically on lesions, but usually no treatment is required. Orf not uncommonly acts as a trigger for an episode of erythema multiforme.

Hand, foot and mouth disease

This disease does not have bovine connotations, nor does it require the placement of trays of disinfectant on the front doorstep and Ministry quarantine regulations. It is produced by Coxsackie virus infection, usually type A16. Small

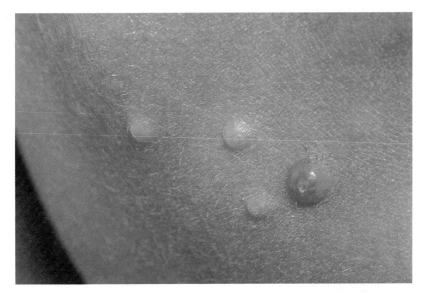

Fig. 3.8. Molluscum contagiosum.

greyish vesicles with a halo of erythema occur on the hands and feet (Fig. 3.10) and the buccal mucosa is studded with erosions resembling aphthous ulcers. The condition resolves within 2 weeks, and no treatment is required.

Herpes simplex

There are two antigenic types of the herpes simplex virus. Type 1 is responsible for the common 'cold sore' on the lips and face, and Type 2 is associated with genital herpes. Neither has rigid territorial demarcation, however, and lesions anywhere on the skin may be caused by either antigenic type.

Primary herpes simplex

Initial contact with the herpes simplex virus usually occurs in early childhood, and any lesions which develop are often so mild that they are not noticed. Occasionally, however, a severe primary herpetic gingivostomatitis occurs, with erosions of the buccal mucosa and lips, and considerable discomfort. Primary cutaneous herpes simplex may also occur, and in an individual suffering from atopic eczema this can be very extensive and may be life-threatening (see below).

Following a primary infection the virus establishes itself in sensory ganglia, and may be triggered to produce recurrent lesions by a variety of stimuli.

Recurrent herpes simplex

Recurrent cold sores on the lips (herpes labialis) are a common problem. Typically the eruption of a group of small vesicles is preceded by a sensation of itching and discomfort in the affected area. The vesicles subsequently burst, the lesion crusts over, and has usually resolved in 10–14 days. The trigger for these

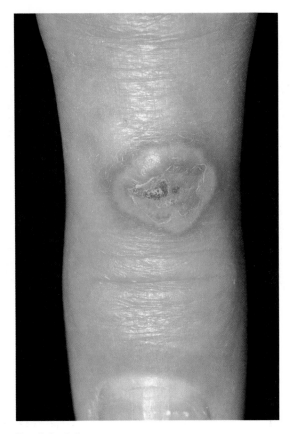

Fig. 3.9. Orf.

episodes is often fever, but exposure to strong sunlight and menses are also recognized precipitants. Sufferers may also claim that anticipation of pleasurable social occasions and holidays triggers cold sores, as they have an irritating habit of appearing just prior to such events. The buttocks are another site for recurrent herpes simplex, and occasionally, as a result of inoculation of the virus into a finger, painful episodes of 'herpetic whitlow' occur. The frequency of episodes of herpes simplex usually gradually declines with advancing years.

Recurrent labial herpes simplex is usually a minor cosmetic inconvenience, and does not require sophisticated therapeutic assault. A little Betadine paint (povidone iodine) will help to prevent secondary bacterial infection, and also has mild antiviral activity. If the lesions are more extensive, then topical Herpid (idoxuridine 5% in dimethyl sulphoxide), or Zovirax cream (acyclovir) can be used for treatment. These agents block viral replication; they are not viricidal, and they are not curative. Labial herpes simplex is a good example of the maxim 'A disease with many remedies has no cure'—suggested therapies are legion, and only the odd cohort or two are of any benefit.

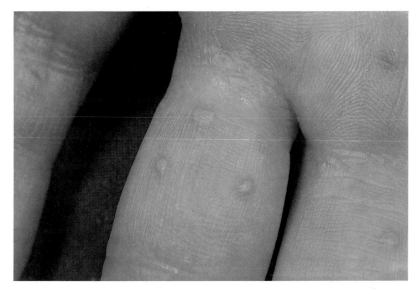

Fig. 3.10. Hand, foot and mouth disease: vesicles on the hand.

Herpes simplex and erythema multiforme

Recurrent herpes simplex can trigger episodes of erythema multiforme. This is a difficult management problem, but the use of a topical antiviral agent as soon as the herpetic lesion begins to develop may shorten its duration, and reduce the likelihood of a subsequent episode of erythema multiforme. The prophylactic use of oral acyclovir has been suggested for severe cases, but the problem recurs as soon as treatment is stopped, and we cannot be certain that long-term acyclovir is free from adverse effects.

Eczema herpeticum (Kaposi's varicelliform eruption)

This is a widespread cutaneous herpes simplex infection which occurs in individuals suffering from atopic eczema. The head and neck are frequently affected, but lesions may spread with alarming rapidity to involve extensive areas of skin. There is associated lymphadenopathy and constitutional upset. A decision about the most appropriate therapy should be based upon whether the lesions are still spreading and whether the patient is systemically unwell. If the lesions are static, and the patient appears well, antiviral chemotherapy is probably unnecessary. If, however, lesions are spreading and the patient is unwell, treatment with intravenous acyclovir (Zovirax i.v.) should be commenced. Most of those affected will be using topical steroids for their eczema, and these should be stopped until the herpes has resolved. Secondary bacterial infection is common, and a systemic antibiotic should be given. Eczema herpeticum is often a recurrent phenomenon, but subsequent episodes tend to be less severe than the primary eruption.

Genital herpes

Genital herpes is a sexually transmitted disease. It may affect the penis, the vulva, the cervix, the perianal area and the rectum. Following the primary episode the virus persists in the presacral ganglia, and like antigenic Type 1 may be triggered to cause recurrent episodes. Genital herpes is potentially more serious in women because of a risk of transmitting the virus to their infants during birth, and the possibility that it may be implicated as a cause of cervical neoplasia. Primary genital herpes in women may be a very uncomfortable illness, with extensive erosions on the vulva, and severe dysuria.

Patients presenting with primary or recurrent genital herpes should be referred to a department of genitourinary medicine for investigation to exclude other sexually transmitted diseases, appropriate management, and expert advice.

Herpes zoster (shingles)

Chicken-pox and herpes zoster are caused by the same virus—the varicella-zoster virus. This is a DNA virus with a size and structure similar to that of the herpes simplex virus. *Shingles* is a distortion of the Latin cingulus, meaning a girdle.

Following an attack of chicken-pox the virus remains dormant in dorsal root ganglia, often for many years, before some stimulus reactivates it and causes an attack of shingles. It is often not obvious what triggering factor is involved, but shingles occurs more frequently in immunosuppressed individuals. It is a disease which principally affects the middle-aged and elderly, but it does occur occasionally in childhood. Anyone who has not suffered from chicken-pox may develop the disease following contact with a case of shingles.

Shingles usually affects a single dermatome, and the thorax and abdomen are the areas most frequently involved. Often the eruption is preceded by a few days pain in the involved area, and this occasionally leads to an incorrect diagnosis of internal pathology. The skin lesions consist of a unilateral band of grouped vesicles on an erythematous base (Fig. 3.11). The contents of the vesicles are initially clear, but become cloudy over a period of a few days. There may be scattered outlying vesicles on the rest of the body, and these outlying lesions tend to be more numerous in the elderly. Numerous outlying vesicles (disseminated zoster) are also a feature of shingles in immunosuppressed individuals, particularly those suffering from Hodgkin's disease or lymphatic leukaemia, and their presence should prompt further investigation of the patient. After a few days the vesicles dry up and form crusts, and in most cases the eruption will have resolved within 2 weeks. However, in the elderly, shingles may produce quite severe erosive changes in the affected area, and these will take considerably longer to heal. Even in the milder cases there is usually some residual scarring in the affected dermatome. The most troublesome aspect of shingles is the persistence of pain after the skin lesions have resolved. This postherpetic neuralgia may be very severe, and is particularly distressing for the elderly.

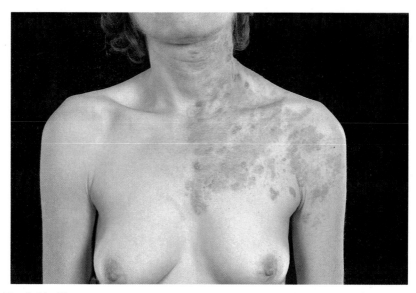

Fig. 3.11. Herpes zoster.

Sacral zoster
Involvement of the sacral segments is commonly complicated by acute retention of urine.

Trigeminal zoster
Herpes zoster may affect any of the divisions of the trigeminal nerve, but the ophthalmic division is most frequently involved (Fig. 3.12). Ocular problems such as conjunctivitis, and occasionally keratitis and/or iridocyclitis are particularly likely to occur if the nasociliary branch of the ophthalmic division is affected.

Involvement of the maxillary division of the trigeminal nerve produces vesicles on the cheek, and unilateral vesicles on the palate.

Motor zoster
Occasionally, in addition to skin lesions in a sensory dermatome, motor fibres originating in the same spinal segment are affected, leading to muscle paralysis and subsequent atrophy.

Treatment of herpes zoster
Most cases of herpes zoster do not require any treatment, but if the patient is seen early in the course of the disease, and lesions are continuing to develop, a topical antiviral agent such as idoxuridine (Herpid) or acyclovir (Zovirax) may shorten the duration of the eruption. In disseminated zoster in the immuno-suppressed, intravenous acyclovir can be life-saving, and it may also be very useful in severe cases of ophthalmic zoster. Patients suffering from ophthalmic

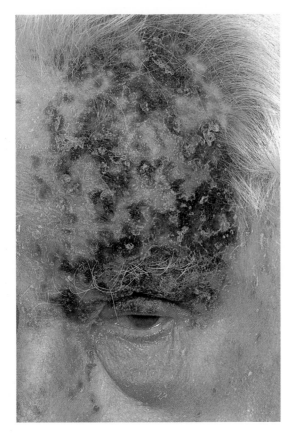

Fig. 3.12. Ophthalmic zoster.

zoster should always be seen by an ophthalmologist to check for ocular involvement.

Effective pain relief is often difficult to achieve in postherpetic neuralgia, and patients with severe discomfort should be referred to a physician experienced in pain-relief techniques.

If patients suffering from shingles require admission to a hospital ward they should be treated in isolation in a side-room. They are a danger to any immunosuppressed patient who has not had chicken-pox, and should not be allowed to mix with other patients. Should a susceptible immunosuppressed patient develop chicken-pox this could be fatal.

Chapter 4
Fungal Infections

The fungi which may cause human disease include the dermatophytes and the yeast-like fungus *Candida albicans* which are responsible for superficial fungal infections confined to the skin and mucous membranes, and others which can invade living tissue to cause deep fungal infections. Deep fungal infections can remain localized (mycetoma) or cause systemic disease (e.g. histoplasmosis).

The dermatophytes are a group of botanically related fungi which are responsible for the so-called 'ringworm' infections. The vegetative phase of dermatophyte fungi consists of septate hyphae which form a branching network (mycelium). *C. albicans* is an organism composed of round or oval cells which divide by budding. Apart from its yeast form it may produce pseudohyphae consisting of numerous cells in a linear arrangement or, in certain circumstances, true septate hyphae.

Dermatophyte infections

It is very easy to become totally confused by the terminology used in fungal infection, and end up not knowing your tinea cruris from your *Trichophyton rubrum*, so don't try to ingest too many Latin names. You can use the term 'ringworm' followed by the location—'of the feet, of the groin, of the scalp,' etc., or if you feel in more classical mood 'tinea' (Latin: a gnawing worm) followed by 'pedis, cruris, capitis' etc. The dermatophyte fungi responsible for skin disease in man are named according to their genus (*Microsporum*, *Trichophyton* and *Epidermophyton*) and their species (e.g. *M. canis*, *T. rubrum*), and they can be distinguished from one another in culture. An experienced dermatologist may be able to suggest that a certain fungus is responsible for a particular case of ringworm, but the only way to establish its identity precisely is by culture.

Some dermatophyte fungi are confined to man (anthropophilic), others principally affect animals (zoophilic) but occasionally infect humans. When animal fungi cause human skin lesions their presence usually provokes a severe inflammatory reaction. Dermatophytes grow only in keratin—the stratum corneum of the skin, the hair, and the nails. Infection is usually indirectly acquired, as a result of contact with keratin debris carrying fungal hyphae; for example, the lady who developed ringworm on the buttocks as a result of her husband's habit of cutting his toe-nails with his feet resting on the lavatory seat.

Tinea pedis (athlete's foot)

This is the commonest of the dermatophyte infections, and usually presents as scaling, itchy areas in the toe-webs, particularly between the fourth and fifth toes (Fig. 4.1). It is usually acquired from contact with infected keratin debris on the

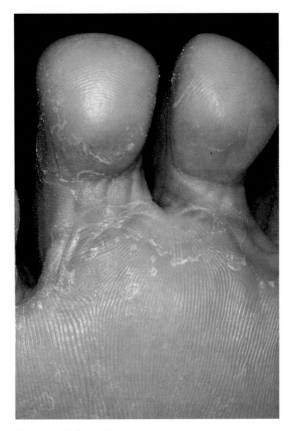

Fig. 4.1. Athlete's foot.

floors of swimming-baths and showers. The condition may spread onto the soles or the dorsa of the feet as areas of scaling erythema. Occasionally athlete's foot follows a pattern of episodic vesicular lesions on the soles of the feet, occurring particularly during warm weather. The feet are frequently asymmetrically involved in fungal infection, in contrast to eczema where the involvement is usually symmetrical.

Tinea cruris

This is a common condition in young adult males. It is rare in women. The clinical picture is characteristic, and should be easy to distinguish from intertrigo, flexural psoriasis or flexural seborrhoeic dermatitis. It is usually symmetrical and affects the inner aspects of the thighs. A scaly, erythematous margin gradually spreads down the thighs (Fig. 4.2) and may extend backwards to involve the perineum and buttocks. The source of the infection is nearly always the patient's feet, so you should always examine the feet for evidence of athlete's foot or fungal nail dystrophy. The fungus is transferred to the groins on the fingers or on towels.

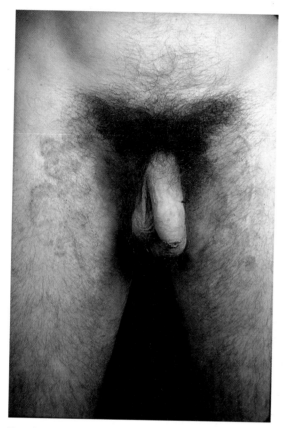

Fig. 4.2. Tinea cruris.

Tinea corporis

The lesions are typically annular, with a scaly inflammatory edge and central clearing (Fig. 4.3). In children the causative organism is usually of animal origin—most frequently from a kitten. In adults the fungus is spread from feet or groins. Tinea corporis is not uncommon in Asian patients, and may be quite extensive.

Tinea manuum

Ringworm on the hand is usually unilateral. On the palm of the hand the appearance is of mild scaling erythema, on the dorsum there is a more obvious inflammatory change with a well-defined edge.

Tinea unguium

Toe-nail fungal dystrophy is very common in adults. It is invariably associated with athlete's foot. The involvement usually starts distally as yellowish streaks in the nail plate (Fig. 4.4), but gradually the whole nail becomes thickened,

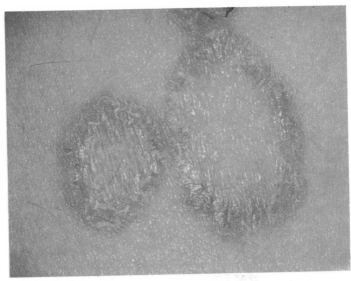

Fig. 4.3. Tinea corporis in a child (*Microsporum canis*–from a cat).

discoloured and friable. The great toe-nails are often the first to be involved, and pressure from footwear on the thickened nails may produce considerable discomfort.

Fungal dystrophy of finger-nails is less common. The changes in the nail plate are similar to those seen in toe-nails. The feet should be examined, because the patient will almost invariably be suffering from athlete's foot and/or tinea of the toe-nails.

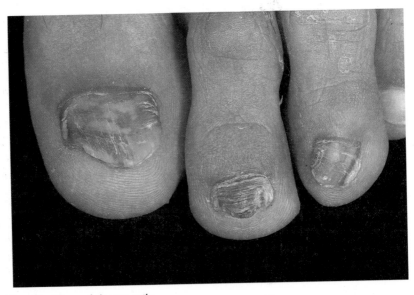

Fig. 4.4. Tinea of the toe-nails.

Tinea capitis

This is a dermatophyte infection of the scalp produced by fungi of the genera *Microsporum* and *Trichophyton*. It is principally a disease of childhood, and is rare in adults. The reason for this is thought to be a change in the fatty acid constituents of sebum around the time of puberty. Postpubertal sebum contains fatty acids which are fungistatic. The principal fungi responsible for scalp ringworm vary in different parts of the world. In Great Britain most cases of childhood scalp ringworm in the indigenous population are the result of *M. canis* infection, usually acquired from cats, and in the USA the usual causative organism is *T. tonsurans*. In the Indian subcontinent the commonest cause is a fungus called *T. violaceum*.

The typical clinical picture is of one or more patches of partial hair loss on an otherwise normal scalp (Fig. 4.5), but occasionally the involvement is more extensive, producing an appearance suggestive of seborrhoeic dermatitis. The affected areas of scalp are scaly, and the hair in these patches is usually broken off just above the surface of the scalp, to produce an irregular stubble. Some species of fungi, for example *M. canis,* fluoresce a brilliant yellow-green under long wavelength UV light (Wood's light)—see Chapter 2.

Kerion (Greek = 'honeycomb')

This is a term applied to a severe inflammatory type of scalp ringworm, usually provoked by the fungus of cattle ringworm, but occasionally occurring with other fungi. The clinical appearance suggests a bacterial infection, with pustules and abscesses (Fig. 4.6), but swabs for bacterial culture are usually negative. When the condition has resolved, there may be areas of permanent hair loss.

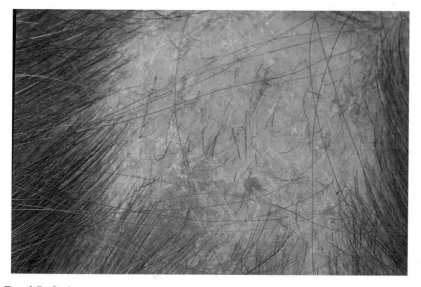

Fig. 4.5. Scalp ringworm.

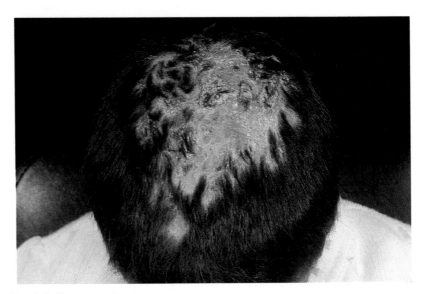

Fig. 4.6. Kerion.

Cattle ringworm

In rural areas it is not uncommon to encounter young farm workers suffering from cattle ringworm—older farmers have usually had the disease, and appear to develop immunity against reinfection. Children who visit farms, or who play in farm fields may pick up the fungus from gates and fences where passing cattle have left keratin debris containing the organism. In adults, the face and forearms are the areas most frequently affected, whereas in children the scalp is the usual site of infection. The fungus provokes a severe inflammatory reaction (Fig. 4.7), which is often misdiagnosed as bacterial in origin.

Tinea incognito

This term is applied to a fungal infection whose appearance has been altered by inappropriate treatment with topical steroid preparations. Topical steroids suppress the inflammatory response to the fungus, and the typical scaly erythematous margin may disappear, leaving an ill-defined area studded with pustules.

'Ide' reactions

Patients suffering from the rather more florid vesicular type of athlete's foot may develop an acute vesiculobullous eruption on the hands 'in sympathy'. The lesions on the hands do not contain fungus. The reaction appears to have an immunological basis, but the exact pathomechanics are not understood. Occasionally, a more generalized maculopapular ide reaction accompanies a fungal infection.

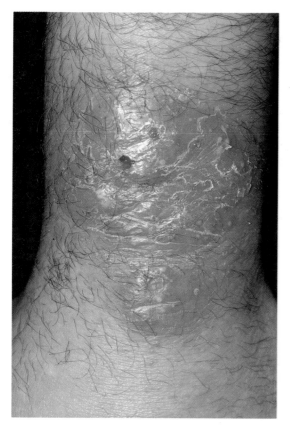

Fig. 4.7. Cattle ringworm on the forearm of a farmer.

Diagnosis

Skin scrapings, nail clippings and plucked hair should be placed on a microscope slide in a few drops of 10% potassium hydroxide, covered with a coverslip, and gently warmed to dissolve the keratin. It is advisable to wait a few minutes for the specimen to 'clear' before examining it under the microscope. A little experience is necessary to distinguish fungal mycelium (Fig. 4.8) from cell walls and intercellular lipid or fragments of cotton sock. Fungal mycelium has the appearance of long rows of railway wagons which branch periodically. Material should also be sent to the mycology laboratory for culture.

In cases of suspected scalp ringworm Wood's light should be shone on the scalp to see if the patches fluoresce, but remember that only a few fungi cause this phenomenon, and the diagnosis can only be confirmed by microscopy of plucked hairs and culture.

Treatment

There are a number of broad-spectrum topical antifungal agents available for the treatment of dermatophyte infections, including miconazole (Daktarin),

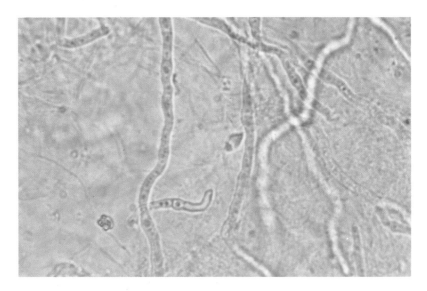

Fig. 4.8. Fungal mycelium.

clotrimazole (Canesten), econazole (Pevaryl) and sulconazole (Exelderm). These can be used when small areas of skin are affected, but if a fungal infection is extensive, it is preferable to employ oral griseofulvin. Athlete's foot is notoriously difficult to clear effectively, probably because of repeated reinfection from footwear, so don't expect any miracles on the feet. Topical agents are not effective in scalp ringworm, and this should always be treated with griseofulvin. For skin and hair infections griseofulvin should be given for a period of 4–6 weeks. In children the dosage is calculated according to the child's weight; in adults the usual daily dose is 500 mg.

Topical therapy for fungal dystrophy of the nails is not effective, although there is now a specially formulated lotion containing tioconazole (Trosyl) which may help in some cases. Nail infections require prolonged treatment with griseofulvin—6 months for finger-nails, and approximately 18 months for toe-nails. Griseofulvin is fungistatic, and is incorporated in nail-plate keratin, forming a barrier to proximal spread of the fungus. Griseofulvin treatment of finger-nails is quite successful, but the cure rate for toe-nails is much lower. Nail growth-rate slows with advancing years, and it is likely that anyone over the age of 60 who takes griseofulvin for toe-nail problems will receive the Queen's telegram before there is any sign of benefit.

Griseofulvin is a safe and effective drug whose introduction in 1959 revolutionized the treatment of dermatophyte infections. Prior to the advent of griseofulvin, scalp ringworm was treated by a process known as X-ray epilation in which the scalp was exposed to a dose of X-rays designed to provoke shedding of the infected hair. Unfortunately, occasional scalps received excessive doses of radiation which produced a permanent scarring alopecia, and a risk of the subsequent development of skin neoplasms in the treated area.

There was even a vogue for the use of the heavy-metal poison thallium in the treatment of scalp ringworm. One effect of thallium is to cause hair shedding, another is to cause death. The vogue for thallium was short-lived, like some of its unfortunate recipients.

Mycetoma (Madura foot)

In certain parts of the world, for example the Indian subcontinent, trauma to the feet may result in the inoculation of certain soil fungi, which produce a chronic infection with abscesses and draining sinuses.

Candida infection

Candidiasis (moniliasis; 'thrush') is a term applied to infections of the skin and mucous membranes by yeast-like fungi of the genus *Candida*, of which *C. albicans* is the principal offending species. *C. albicans* is a normal commensal of the human digestive tract, where it exists in balance with the bacterial flora. In its commensal role, *Candida* is present as budding yeasts. In a pathogenic role, budding and mycelial forms are usually present. It is kept in check by the normal defence systems of the host, and by the gut flora, and only becomes pathogenic when situations favourable to its multiplication arise. A number of factors predispose to candidiasis, including topical and systemic steroid therapy, immune suppression of any aetiology, whether therapeutic or associated with disease (e.g. lymphoma, HIV infection), broad-spectrum antibiotics, diabetes mellitus, and the apposition of areas of skin producing a warm, moist environment.

The diagnosis of candidiasis can be confirmed by culture of swabs taken from the affected areas.

Buccal mucosal candidiasis

The characteristic clinical appearance in this condition is of white, curd-like plaques adhering to the buccal mucosa. If these are scraped off, the underlying mucosa is inflamed and friable. Buccal candidiasis is common in patients treated with broad-spectrum antibiotics. It may be treated with nystatin oral suspension, amphotericin lozenges (Fungilin lozenges) or miconazole gel (Daktarin oral gel).

Angular cheilitis (perlèche)

As we age, the vertical dimensions of the face gradually diminish, a process significantly accelerated by the extraction of all the teeth! This leads to the development of deep grooves at the angles of the mouth. Saliva is drawn into these grooves by capillary action, and salivary enzymes macerate the skin, producing sore, moist areas at the corners of the mouth (Fig. 4.9). *Candida* from the mouth multiplies in these conditions, and exacerbates the problem. Most patients presenting with this problem are denture wearers, and their angular cheilitis may be helped by modification of the dentures. The topical application of nystatin cream, or an imidazole (clotrimazole, miconazole, econazole) will also help. Occasionally angular cheilitis is a feature of iron

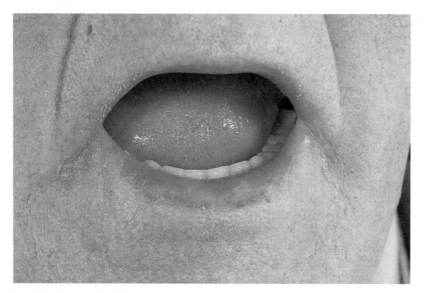

Fig. 4.9. Angular cheilitis.

deficiency or vitamin B_{12} deficiency, and it is therefore advisable to perform a full blood count in anyone suffering from this problem.

Chronic paronychia

This condition is a chronic inflammatory process affecting the proximal nail fold and nail matrix. *C. albicans* plays a major pathogenic role in chronic paronychia, but bacteria may also be involved. This condition, however, is quite distinct from an acute staphylococcal paronychia, in which there is a short history, severe discomfort, and ample production of laudable green pus. The typical clinical appearance in chronic paronychia is of thickening and erythema of the proximal nail fold ('bolstering'), and loss of the cuticle (Fig. 4.10). There is often an associated nail dystrophy. Chronic paronychia occurs predominantly in those whose hands are repeatedly immersed in water—housewives, barmaids, florists, fishmongers.

Treatment consists of advice to keep the hands as dry as possible by wearing cotton-lined rubber or PVC gloves when working, and topical anti-*Candida* therapy.

Balanitis/vulvovaginitis

C. balanitis is an affliction of the uncircumcised. Small white patches or eroded areas are present on the foreskin and glans. Predisposing factors are poor penile hygiene, and diabetes mellitus. *C. balanitis* may be a recurrent problem if a sexual partner has *C. vaginitis*.

C. vulvovaginitis presents with a creamy vaginal discharge and itchy erythema of the vulva. Pregnancy, oral contraceptives and diabetes mellitus are predisposing factors.

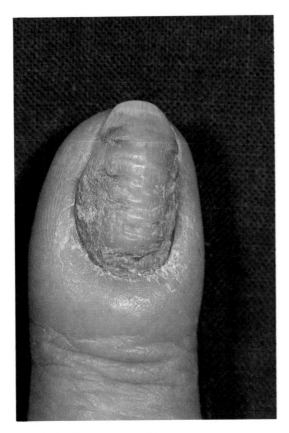

Fig. 4.10. Chronic paronychia.

Balanitis and vulvitis should be treated with a topical anti-*Candida* preparation, and there are several products available to treat vaginal candidiasis.

Don't forget to test the urine for sugar in anyone with C. balanitis or vulvovaginitis.

Intertrigo

Interigo is a term applied to inflammation and maceration of skin in areas where two skin surfaces are in apposition—groins, axillae, submammary regions, beneath an abdominal apron of fat. Obesity and poor hygiene are contributory factors. *Candida* superinfection is often present, and can be recognized clinically by the presence of creamy 'satellite' pustules at the margins of the affected areas. The pustules are easily ruptured, leaving a tiny collarette of scale, and the coalescence of many of these lesions gives a characteristic scalloped edge to the area of intertrigo.

Combination therapy with a preparation containing an anti-*Candida* agent and hydrocortisone is usually effective in keeping the condition under control:

Nystaform HC cream (nystatin, chlorhexidine, hydrocortisone); Daktacort cream (miconazole, hydrocortisone); or Canesten HC cream (clotrimazole, hydrocortisone). However, it usually recurs because the only long-term solution in many cases is a radically restructured anatomy.

Pityriasis (tinea) versicolor

This is a common condition in young adults caused by yeast-like organisms (*Pityrosporum* species), which are normal skin commensals present in pilo sebaceous follicles. It would appear that an alteration in the microenvironment of these organisms, in affected individuals, encourages them to multiply and extend onto the surface of the skin. Most affected individuals are perfectly well otherwise, but diabetics and patients taking systemic steroids have a higher incidence of this condition.

On a non-pigmented skin the lesions of pityriasis versicolor are light-brown macules with a fine surface scale, and occur predominantly on the trunk (Fig. 4.11). They are usually asymptomatic. On a pigmented skin, particularly that of a Caucasian after sunbathing, the typical appearance is of patchy hypopigmentation.

The diagnosis can be confirmed by microscopic examination of skin scrapings in a mixture of 10% potassium hydroxide and Parker Quink ink (Fig. 4.12), when characteristic clumps of round spores and short, stubby hyphae can be seen ('spaghetti and meat balls').

A simple and effective treatment is the use of topical selenium sulphide in the form of Selsun shampoo. This can be left on the skin for a few minutes during bathing, and will usually clear the organism in 2–3 weeks. The broad-spectrum topical antifungal agents such as miconazole, clotrimazole,

Ketoconazole 400mg tablet single dose 5/92.

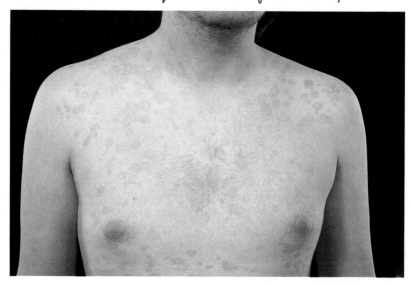

Fig. 4.11. Pityriasis versicolor.

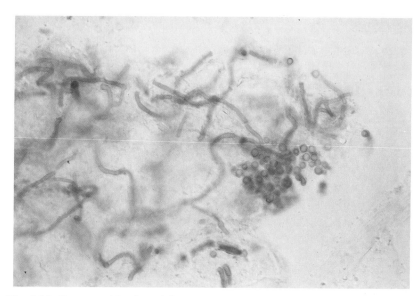

Fig. 4.12. Spores and hyphae of *Pityrosporum* in pityriasis versicolor.

and econazole are also effective against this organism—griseofulvin, however, is not. Tinea versicolor has a marked tendency to recur, and treatment may have to be repeated at intervals. Hypopigmented areas may take considerable time to re-pigment, and their persistence should not be taken as evidence of treatment failure.

Chapter 5
Ectoparasite Infections

Scabies

There's a squeak of pure delight from a matey little mite,
As it tortuously tunnels in the skin,
Singing furrow, folly furrow, come and join me in my burrow,
And we'll view the epidermis from within.

(Guy's Acarus)

Aetiology

Scabies is caused by the mite *Sarcoptes scabiei* (Greek = 'flesh cutter'), and is acquired by close physical contact with someone else suffering from the disease—sexual contact is often implicated, but prolonged hand holding is probably a frequent means of spread. Any age group may be affected, but it is commoner in children and young adults. Transient contact is not sufficient for spread, and doctors and nurses coming in contact with ordinary cases of scabies should not be afraid of acquiring the disease.

On the skin of the host the female scabies mite burrows in the stratum corneum, and after fertilization by the male, she begins to lay eggs in the burrow behind her. Male scabies mites have but one function in life, and after the chase and the consummation they expire. Initially the host is unaware of the mining activity in the epidermis, but after a period of some 4–6 weeks hypersensitivity to mite faeces develops, and itching begins. Thereafter, life for the mites becomes hazardous as burrows will be excoriated and mites and eggs destroyed. In this way the host keeps the mite population in check, and in most individuals suffering from scabies the average number of adult female mites on the skin is no more than a dozen.

Clinical features

The patient suffering from scabies complains of itching, which is characteristically worse at night. Scabies should be considered in anyone presenting with this history.

There are two principal types of skin lesion in scabies—burrows, and the scabies 'rash' (Table 5.1). Burrows are found principally on the hands and feet—the sides of the fingers and toes, the web-spaces, the wrists, and the insteps of the feet. In infants, burrows are often present on the palms of the hands and soles of the feet, and may also be present on the trunk. Each

Table 5.1. Scabies: clinical features

Primary lesions	Secondary lesions
Burrows	Excoriations
Scabies 'rash'	Eczematization
	Secondary infection

burrow is several millimetres long, often tortuous, faintly brown in colour, and frequently there is mild erythema of the surrounding skin (Fig. 5.1). Burrows also occur on the male genitalia, usually surmounting an inflammatory papule, and the presence of these lesions in this situation is pathognomonic of scabies. If scabies is suspected in a male, the genitalia should always be examined.

The 'rash' of scabies is an eruption of tiny inflammatory papules grouped on the axillary folds, around the umbilicus, and on the thighs (Fig. 5.2). The aetiology of these papules is not known with certainty, but they are thought to occur as a reaction to burrowing immature mites.

In addition to these primary skin lesions, the clinical picture may be confused by the presence of secondary changes such as excoriations, eczematization and secondary bacterial infection. In certain parts of the world, secondary infection of scabies lesions with nephritogenic streptococci may result in cases of poststreptococcal glomerulonephritis.

Diagnosis

Absolute confirmation of the diagnosis can only be made by demonstrating the mite or eggs microscopically. In order to do this, burrows must be found, and this usually requires some experience. Look carefully, in good light, at the hands and feet. A magnifying glass may be of some help, but the myopic amongst us simply discard our spectacles. Once a burrow, or suspected burrow, has been identified, it should be gently scraped off the skin with the edge of a blunt scalpel—dermatologists often use an instrument with a slightly curved blade known as a 'banana' scalpel for this task. The burrow and its contents should be placed on a microscope slide with a few drops of 10% potassium hydroxide,

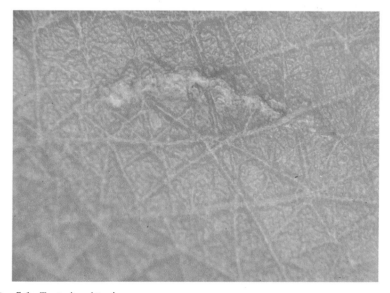

Fig. 5.1. Typical scabies burrow.

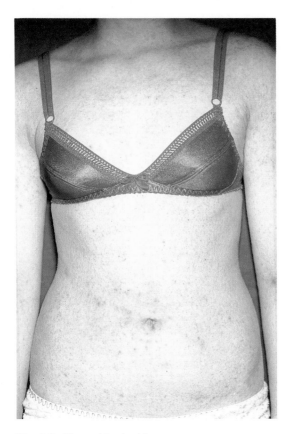

Fig. 5.2. The scabies 'rash',

covered with a coverslip, and examained under the microscope. The presence of mites, eggs, or even eggshells confirms the diagnosis (Fig. 5.3).

An alternative to the banana-scalpel routine is what might be referred to as the 'winkle-picker' technique. At the end of each intact burrow is a tiny vesicle, adjacent to which the female mite is burrowing. If the vesicle is opened with a needle, the tip of which is gently moved around within it, the mite can often be removed on the end of the needle.

Do not attempt to scrape lesions on the penis—the proximity of a banana scalpel to the nether regions leads to understandable apprehension, and is in any case rarely rewarded by the demonstration of mites.

Treatment

Scabies is treated by eating young alligators and washing the skin with urine.
(Mexican Folk Medicine)

It is most important to explain to patients precisely how to use their treatment, and written explanatory treatment sheets are very useful for this purpose. All family members, and close physical contacts of an affected individual should be

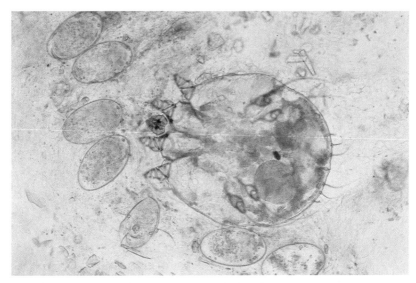

Fig. 5.3. Scabies mite and eggs in potassium hydroxide preparation.

treated simultaneously. The topical therapy should be applied with a two-inch paint-brush from the neck to the toes. Itching does not resolve immediately following treatment, but will improve gradually over a period of 2–3 weeks as the stratum corneum, containing the allergenic mite faeces, is shed. A topical antipruritic such as Eurax hydrocortisone cream (crotamiton 10% and hydrocortisone 0.25%) can be used on residual itchy areas. It is not necessary to 'disinfect' clothing and soft furnishings—laundering of underwear and nightclothes is all that is required.

Suggested treatment regimes

Benzyl benzoate emulsion Two or three applications in a 24-h period are usually sufficient. On the evening of day 1 apply the emulsion from the neck to the toes. Allow to dry, then apply a second coat. The following morning apply a third coat, and then wash off the benzyl benzoate on the evening of day 2. Treatment is then complete, and this should be stressed to the patient, because benzyl benzoate is an irritant, and repeated use will produce an irritant dermatitis.

Gamma-benzene hexachloride lotion (Quellada lotion) One application from the neck to the toes is sufficient. The lotion is left on the skin for 12–24 h, and then washed off.

Monosulfiram (Tetmosol) Before application Tetmosol should be diluted with two to three parts of water. The dilute solution is then applied from neck to toes, and washed off after 24 h.

Aqueous malathion (Derbac-M liquid) One application from the neck to the toes, washed off after 24 h.

Scabies mites do not burrow on the head and neck, except in infants, and it is not necessary to treat these areas.

Treatment of infants and young children

Benzyl benzoate is an irritant, and should be diluted to half-strength if being used to treat babies. Any of the other regimes mentioned above can be used in the treatment of young children, although there is some debate about γ-benzene hexachloride as there have been reports of transient neurological problems following its use on infants. The experience of most dermatologists is that it is safe if used correctly.

If burrows are present on the head and neck area in babies, these can be treated with topical Eurax (crotamiton 10%) cream.

Norwegian (crusted) scabies

This is an uncommon type of scabies in which enormous numbers of mites are present in crusted lesions on the skin. It is called Norwegian scabies because it was originally described in Norwegian lepers—the mite is exactly the same as that causing ordinary scabies. Mites are present in such huge numbers because of an altered host response to their presence. Norwegian scabies may develop when itching is not perceived because of mental abnormality, sensory loss from neurological disorders, or when the hypersensitivity response to the parasites is suppressed. Physical incapacity may also so limit the ability to scratch that the mite population gradually multiplies unchecked. Norwegian scabies occurs in the mentally defective, particularly patients with Down's syndrome, those immobilized by hemiparesis, quadriparesis or severe arthropathy, and patients who are immunosuppressed, either as a result of disease (e.g. lymphoma, AIDS) or treatment of disease (e.g. systemic steroids, organ transplantation).

The skin lesions in Norwegian scabies contain thousands of mites and eggs, and these are shed into the environment of the patient on flakes of keratin. Anyone coming into contact with such an individual is at considerable risk of developing ordinary scabies, and undiagnosed cases of Norwegian scabies are often responsible for outbreaks of scabies amongst the personnel of hospitals and residential accommodation for the elderly.

Clinical features

The hands and feet are usually encased in a heavy, fissured crust, and areas of crusting may be present on other parts of the body. The changes may resemble psoriatic scaling or a hyperkeratotic eczema, and this is why the diagnosis may be missed. Burrows are usually impossible to identify in the crusted areas, but may be found on less severely affected parts of the body.

Treatment

The patient should be isolated, and nurses responsible for the patient's care should wear gowns and gloves. All nursing and medical staff who have had contact with the patient, and all other patients sharing the same accommodation should be treated with a topical scabicide.

Norwegian scabies responds to the same treatments used in ordinary scabies, but several applications of a scabicide are usually required to eradicate the problem.

Pediculosis

Head lice (Pediculus humanus capitis)

Her ladyship said when I went to her house,
That she did not esteem me three skips of a louse;
I freely forgave what the dear creature said,
For ladies will talk of what runs in their head.
(Theodore Hook)

Head lice are wingless insects which live on the scalp, and feed on blood. Adult head lice are approximately 2–3 mm in length. They are acquired by head-to-head contact with another individual harbouring the parasite. Medical entomologists do not consider that fomites, such as caps, brushes and combs, are responsible for transmission of the head louse. In the past, head-louse infection was principally a problem of the lower classes in large industrial conurbations, but in recent years the head louse has climbed the social ladder and has become a problem of the middle classes. Fortunately, the incidence of head-louse infection is now declining.

The adult female louse lays eggs which she cements to hair shafts (Fig. 5.4). The eggs are laid close to the surface of the scalp and will have hatched before the hair has grown more than a few millimetres. The eggs are flesh-coloured

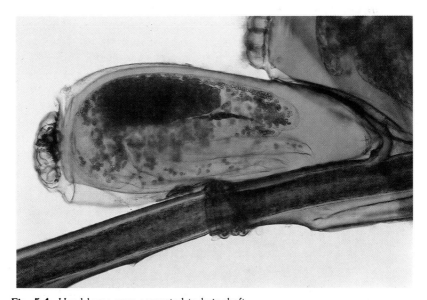

Fig. 5.4. Head louse eggs cemented to hair shaft.

and are difficult to see, but once the louse nymph has emerged the empty egg-case (nit) is more easily seen.

Clinical features

Itching is the main symptom of head louse infection. Nits tend to be more numerous in the occipital region of the scalp and above the ears. Occasionally flakes of dandruff or keratin casts may be mistaken for nits clinically, but the distinction is obvious if the material is examined microscopically. Adult lice and nymphs will be found without difficulty in the heavier infections (Fig. 5.5). Impetigo may occur as a result of inoculation of staphylococci into the skin during scratching—the term 'nitwit' is derived from the substandard performance of children who had large head louse populations, secondary skin sepsis, and probably also anaemia, and were chronically unwell as a result.

Treatment

It is principally thanks to the efforts of the School Nursing Service and a few medical entomologists that the incidence of head-louse infection has fallen to such a low level in recent years. The insecticides malathion and carbaryl are

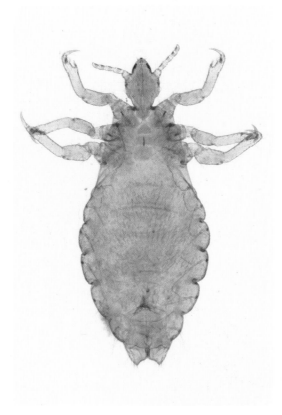

Fig. 5.5. The head louse.

used to treat head-louse infection in Great Britain. Both are efficient pediculi-cides and ovicides, and there are several proprietary preparations available (Table 5.2). Malathion is adsorbed onto keratin, a process which takes about 6 h, and confers a residual protective effect against reinfection which lasts for approximately 6 weeks. Carbaryl is not adsorbed in this way, and does not confer any residual protective effect. Prioderm lotion, Derbac-M liquid and Carylderm lotion should be left on the scalp for 12 h before being washed out. Suleo-M and Suleo-C are marketed as 'rapid' treatments for head lice, to be washed out after 2 h. Both malathion and carbaryl are degraded by heat, and should be stored in a cool environment. After the application of these lotions the hair should be allowed to dry naturally, not with the aid of a hot-air hair-dryer, and certainly not in front of the fire—most of these preparations are alcohol-based and highly inflammable. Treatment should be repeated after 7–10 days to deal with any louse nymphs emerging from surviving eggs. All family contacts should also be treated. It is not necessary to remove nits with a nit comb, except for cosmetic reasons.

Don't use insecticidal shampoos for the definitive treatment of head lice—these expose the insects to a low concentration of insecticide, and carry the risk of encouraging the emergence of insecticide resistance in the lice.

Body lice (Pediculus humanus humanus)

> The louse
> Has very little 'nous',
> Its only pursuit
> Is the hirsute.
> (I. Kenvyn Evans)

The body, or clothing louse is a parasite of poverty and poor hygiene. It lives, and lays its eggs in clothing, and only moves onto the body to feed on blood. It flourishes in an environment which is warm, and as little disturbed as possible. It is still common in the poorer countries of the world, but in an affluent society its usual hosts are tramps and down-and-outs who have only one set of clothes which are never removed or cleaned. An individual who regularly changes clothing and maintains a reasonable standard of hygiene will never be a host to body lice because they will not survive being removed from the warmth of the body, and the rigours of laundering and ironing. Body lice are vectors of epidemic typhus, which has been responsible for millions of deaths over the centuries.

Table 5.2. Proprietary preparations for head louse treatment

Malathion:
   Prioderm lotion
   Derbac-M liquid
   Suleo-M
Carbaryl:
   Carylderm lotion
   Suleo-C

Clinical features

Body lice usually provoke itching, and their host is often covered in excoriations. The itching appears to be the result of an acquired hypersensitivity to louse saliva. Occasional individuals seem to have little or no itching, and their louse populations may be very numerous. The socks in Fig. 5.6 belonged to a patient who was teeming with lice, but had no skin lesions of any significance. If you suspect body louse infection there is no point in searching the patient for lice—you may be lucky and find the odd one at lunch, but it is the clothing you should examine.

Treatment

All the patient requires is a bath. Underclothing should be laundered, and any lice and eggs in the outer clothing will be killed by 15 min in a tumble-dryer.

Crab lice (Pthirus pubis)

It's no good standing on the seat
The crabs in here can jump ten feet.
If you think that's rather high,
Go next door, the buggers fly!
                    (Toilet graffito)

The crab louse, or pubic louse, in spite of the above allegation of contagion from hinged lavatory components, is probably most frequently transmitted by direct physical contact with an infected individual. It has always been considered a rather sedentary louse, but recent studies suggest that when its host is sleeping, the crab louse becomes quite active. It is a louse adapted to living in hair of a particular density. Scalp hair follicles are too densely packed for its comfort, but pubic, axillary, beard, and eyelash hair are perfectly acceptable to

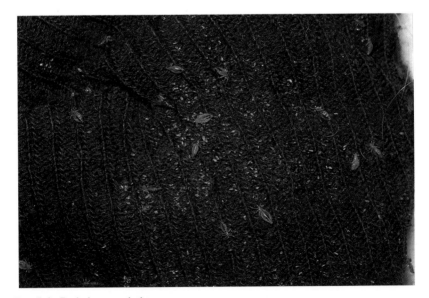

Fig. 5.6. Body lice on clothing.

it, and in the extremely hairy male it may be found widely distributed over the trunk and limbs. The crab louse is so named because of its squat shape and powerful claws, resembling a crab's pincers (Fig. 5.7), with which it grasps hair very firmly. Female crab lice, like head lice, stick their eggs to hair shafts with a cement material.

Clinical features

Itching is the symptom which draws the host's attention to these little passengers. Self-examination then usually reveals the reason for the itch, and the doctor is often presented with a small envelope, or folded piece of paper containing specimens. Always open the folded paper carefully, as it has a tendency to flick the crab lice in all directions, leaving one anxiously awaiting signs of personal contamination for weeks thereafter.

Lice are usually visible on the pubic area or in the axillae, but sometimes their eggs, which are a brown colour, are easier to see. Where the parasites are very numerous the underclothes may be speckled with spots of altered blood excreted by the lice. Lice on the eyelids festoon the lashes with their eggs (Fig. 5.8).

Treatment

Any of the insecticide preparations used in the treatment of head lice may also be used to eradicate crab lice. However, alcohol is rather irritant on the scrotum, and it is preferable to use Derbac-M liquid (malathion 0.5%) which has an aqueous base, and is non-irritant (Derbac is an anagram of de-crab). Always remember to treat the axillae, and hairy males should be anointed from neck to toes. Sexual contacts should also be treated. The treatment should be repeated after an interval of 7–10 days.

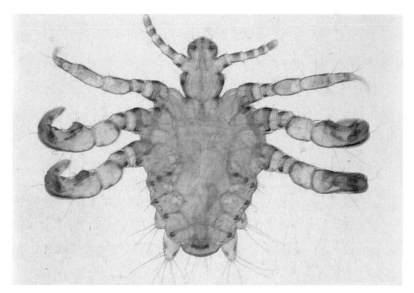

Fig. 5.7. The crab louse.

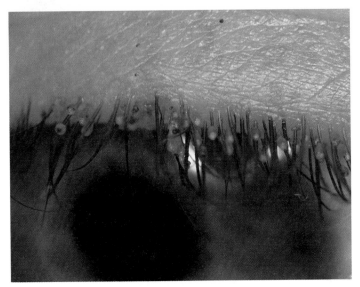

Fig. 5.8. Crab louse eggs on the eyelashes.

Eyelash infestation should also be treated with the aqueous-based Derbac-M liquid smeared over the lids and lashes. The other available insecticide preparations will irritate the eyes.

Papular urticaria

Usually referred to as 'heat bumps' by patients, papular urticaria is the typical response to the bites of a number of arthropods, including biting flies, mosquitoes, mites, fleas and bed-bugs. The lesions of papular urticaria are small urticated papules (Fig. 5.9), often surmounted by a tiny vesicle, and they are so itchy that their tops are rapidly excoriated. They arise as a result of a hypersensitivity response to antigens in the arthropods' saliva. Not everyone reacts to these antigens, and in those who do react tolerance is often acquired after a variable length of time.

Fleas

May the fleas of a thousand camels infest your armpits!
(Arab curse)

Perhaps the commonest cause of papular urticaria acquired in the home environment is that due to flea bites. It is not the human flea (*Pulex irritans*) which is responsible, as this is no longer encountered in Great Britain on humans, but fleas whose natural hosts are household pets. A familiar clinical picture is of multiple lesions around the ankles of the ladies of the household (Fig. 5.10). Men are rarely affected because socks and trousers deny the fleas access to the ankles.

Cats and dogs are perambulating quadripedal 'meals-on-wheels' for the fleas, and although adult fleas can be found on the animals it is really the

Fig. 5.9. Papular urticaria.

household which is infested. Flea eggs are not sticky, and when laid by fleas feeding on an animal they drop out of the coat into the surroundings—the cat-basket, the carpet, the counterpane or the vicar's lap. So the house should be treated, as well as the pets therein. One of the best preparations to deal with flea infestation is a combination of a standard insecticide, permethrin, with methoprene, a synthetic equivalent of an insect growth regulatory hormone, in an aerosol can (Acclaim Plus). The methoprene blocks the metamorphosis of flea larvae into adults. This should be sprayed around the carpets and soft furnishings, and the animals' sleeping areas, and will confer protection against flea infestation for 4 months.

Occasionally bird fleas will gain access to homes from nests under the eaves, and may be responsible for more extensive lesions of papular urticaria.

Bed-bugs (Cimex lectularius)

The butterfly has wings of gold,
The firefly wings of flame,
The bed-bug has no wings at all,
But he gets there just the same.

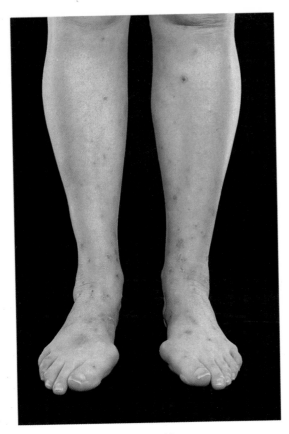

Fig. 5.10. Flea bites on the ankles.

Perhaps this rhyme relates to the, probably inaccurate, tale that attempts to stop bed bugs crawling up bed legs at night by placing the legs in bowls of water can be frustrated by the cunning bugs climbing the walls, crossing the ceiling, and dropping on the occupants of the bed from above.

Bed-bugs are not the most appealing of creatures. They live in dilapidated housing behind peeling wallpaper and rotten skirting boards, and emerge an hour or so before dawn to feed on the sleeping occupants of bedrooms. They feed on blood, and although the process of feeding does not cause the host any pain, a reaction to the bites of the bugs usually results in papular urticaria or bullous lesions. These insects are 5–6 mm long, dark brown in colour, and can move quite rapidly. Fortunately, bed-bug infestation of houses is now an uncommon occurrence, but if it is suspected the local Environmental Health Department should be asked to inspect the property and deal with any infestation.

Animal mites

Human contact with animals suffering from sarcoptic mange may result in the development of scattered, itchy papules, often on areas coming into contact with the animals—for example the abdomen and thighs if a mangy dog sits on its owner's lap. It is extremely rare for these animal mites to establish themselves on humans, though there have been a few reported cases.

Dogs, cats and rabbits are the natural hosts of Cheyletiella mites, and these may cause skin lesions in humans. Man's best friend is the usual culprit. On the animal, the mites provoke a heavy scurf over the back ('walking dandruff'), but hardly bother it otherwise. On the owner, itchy papules appear principally on the abdomen, but occasionally also on the thighs and arms—sites of contact with the animal. The diagnosis can be confirmed by taking combings from the animal's coat and demonstrating the mite microscopically. Once the animal has been treated by a veterinary practitioner the human skin lesions resolve spontaneously.

Bird mites may gain access to houses from nests under the eaves, via windows and ventilation grilles, and can cause itchy papular lesions on the occupants.

Ticks

Ticks are very common in Great Britain, particularly in wooded areas where there are deer populations. They feed on blood, and their barbed mouthparts are held in the skin of the host during feeding by a protein cement material. If a tick is pulled off the skin abruptly, its mouthparts may be left in situ, and will provoke a foreign-body reaction.

Ticks are vectors of Lyme disease which is caused by the spirochaete *Borrelia burgdorferi*. Lyme disease (named after the town in Connecticut where its association with ticks was first discovered) affects the skin, joints, central nervous system, and the heart. It responds to treatment with penicillin or tetracyclines.

The classical method of tick removal is the application of a lighted cigarette to its rear end—anything will let go under this stimulus, but it is now becoming more difficult to find anyone with a cigarette to participate in this manoeuvre. Probably the best method of tick removal is to grasp it as close to the skin as possible, and exert gentle continuous traction.

Chapter 6
Acne, Acneiform Eruptions and Rosacea

Out, damned spot! Out, I say!
(William Shakespeare, *Macbeth* V.I. (38))

This chapter deals with a number of disorders which give rise to papules and pustules, often known in the vernacular as 'spots' or 'zits'. Some of these conditions appear aetiologically related to each other and can properly be called variants of acne (probably a corruption of the Greek word *akme* = 'a point'), while others produce lesions closely or superficially resembling 'true' acne: acneiform disorders and rosacea.

We shall begin by looking at the acne 'family':
Acne vulgaris
  Classical
  Infantile and juvenile onset
  Late-onset
  Severe (acne conglobata/nodulocystic)
  With systemic symptoms (acne fulminans)
Secondary acne
  Endocrine-associated
  Medicaments
  Oils
  Chloracne
    Hidradenitis suppurativa

Acne vulgaris and its variants

Acne vulgaris is a very common condition: about 80% of us develop a tendency to spottiness at some stage of our lives. This is usually during adolescence and early adult life but the onset may be much earlier or much later. In a few, the lesions of acne are induced by underlying endocrinological abnormalities, such as the polycystic ovary syndrome. Acne may be very mild indeed but at its most severe acne vulgaris exhibits gross changes which are extremely unsightly. This end of the spectrum is sometimes accorded a separate designation: acne conglobata.

However, these variants have much more in common with one another than the differences which appear to distinguish them. We shall therefore discuss acne vulgaris as a single entity, but pointing out the differences in the subtypes listed above, where they arise.

Clinical features

Age of onset and course

Most acne sufferers experience their first problems in adolescence, although there are exceptions to this (see below). It may follow close on the heels of the first signs of puberty or may be delayed by some months or years. It is important to note that the lesions of acne vary considerably with time. For example, most patients notice marked fluctuations in the number of spots and in the severity of the inflammation. In girls, there is often a premenstrual flare and in both sexes the condition frequently deteriorates at times of stress.

The severity of acne tends to increase for the first 2 or 3 years after onset before gradually settling and, in the majority, disappearing altogether. The peak of severity is usually earlier in girls than in boys. Unfortunately for some, the time course may be much more prolonged, with lesions continuing to develop well into the late twenties and beyond. There are also two groups of patients in whom true acne develops well outside the adolescent period:

Infantile/juvenile acne Typical acne lesions are occasionally seen in infants and children. The problems usually begin when the child is 3–12 months old and last for 4 or 5 years. This is mostly a disorder of boys. Although the early onset lesions subside, adolescence often brings a severe recrudescence. Endocrine abnormalities are very rarely found but should be considered, especially in a girl if there are signs of virilism.

Late-onset acne Some women develop typical lesions of acne in their 30s and 40s. There are often premenstrual exacerbations. Endocrinological investigation is generally unrewarding.

The psychological impact of acne

There is no doubt that acne can make life really miserable and the fact that it has a predilection for the teens and 20s means that it affects those who are least well-equipped emotionally to cope with it. The face is prominently involved and during adolescence the face assumes increasing importance as a means of projecting an attractive image. At the time when acne strikes the individual is beginning to become aware of the drive to form major relationships outside the family and the close circle of same-sex friends: pair-bonding is the new game.

It is during this formative period that acne wreaks most of its havoc. It is important to realize that the psychological impact of acne is not necessarily related to the absolute degree of severity of the disease. A young sufferer may spend just as long staring miserably at him/herself in the mirror when there are only a few spots as when there are hundreds.

Physical signs

Site and distribution   The lesions of acne have a characteristic distribution. The major sites of activity are: the face, any part of which may be involved; the neck, especially posteriorly; the upper back; the anterior chest, in an inverted 'V' from the shoulders to the xiphisternum; the shoulders; the ears. In the most severely affected individuals lesions may extend down the arms and the whole of the central back may be affected, with lesions even extending onto the buttocks.

The appearance of the skin The first physical sign to note in acne is that the skin of the face and upper trunk becomes very greasy (Fig. 6.1). This is due to a marked increase in the production of sebum. This happens normally at puberty, but is usually particularly pronounced in those with bad acne. Overproduction of sebum involves the scalp too, resulting in very greasy hair. Greasiness alone may be sufficiently severe for the patient to seek advice. This is not a feature of the prepubertal onset.

The individual lesions of acne A cardinal feature of acne is that it is a polymorphic disorder. Most sufferers develop several different types of lesion at any one time and the presence of such variability is an important pointer towards the diagnosis. Acne sufferers generally have several of the following lesions:

Comedones
Papules and pustules
Nodules and cysts
Scars

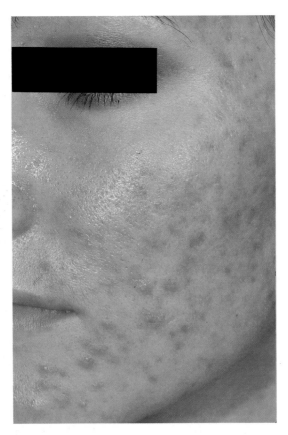

Fig. 6.1. This girl's face shows the typical greasy skin of the acne sufferer, in addition to papules and pustules.

Comedones (singular: comedo) Although some dispute the importance of the comedone in the pathogenesis of the inflammatory lesions of acne, their presence is a very important diagnostic aid. There are two types of comedo: the closed (or 'whitehead') and the open (or 'blackhead').

Closed comedones can be felt better than seen. They are very small papules, often with a central point or elevation (Fig. 6.2). They may occur anywhere in the distribution described above but are often most numerous across the forehead and on the cheeks. There is usually little or no inflammation.

Open comedones (blackheads) are very familiar. They consist of dilated, blocked hair follicles with a black dot at the mouth. It is not entirely clear what the black dot is due to.

Some sufferers have many hundreds of open comedones. In severe acne burnt out inflammatory lesions may leave multiheaded blackheads ('polyporous comedones'), particularly on the shoulders and upper trunk. Blackheads are a useful diagnostic aid since they are virtually pathognomonic of acne in the younger patient (although advanced solar damage may also result in blackhead formation).

In some patients, comedones are virtually the only lesions present.

Papules and pustules These are relatively superficial lesions. The majority of patients with acne develop at least some papules and pustules. Some have hundreds. Lesions of this kind consist of small red spots or pustules on a red base (see Fig. 6.1) and may be itchy or painful. Papules frequently become pustular during the course of their evolution. They develop rapidly, often over a few hours, and it is not unusual for the patient to wake in the morning to find

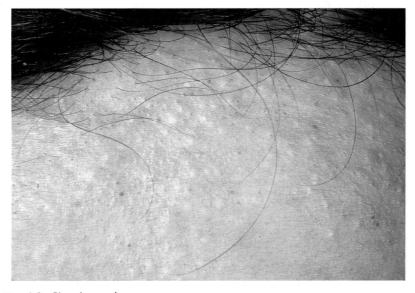

Fig. 6.2. Closed comedones.

several brand-new spots. They resolve over the course of a few days. New lesions may arise in exactly the same site on many occasions.

Nodules and cysts   As the degree and depth of the inflammation increases, so does the size of the visible and palpable lesions. Deep-seated nodules and cysts are less common than papules and pustules, but many acne patients develop a few. Some have large numbers. As pustules accompany papules, so cysts may accompany nodules. In some patients nodules and cysts predominate (Fig. 6.3 (a), (b)). It is these individuals to whom the terms 'acne conglobata' or 'nodulocystic acne' are applied.

The lesions in this severe form of the disease are often extremely uncomfortable and usually last much longer than more superficial changes. Some become chronic and may even result in permanent epidermoid cyst formation.

Scars   The final common pathway for all the inflammatory processes seen in acne is scarring. By no means all lesions leave scars, but many do and these remain as a lifetime's legacy of adolescent anguish. The characteristic patterns are small, dimpled or 'ice-pick' scars, but more severe disease can leave gross scarring with atrophic areas (Fig. 6.4) or even keloid formation.

Systemic symptoms (acne fulminans)

Very occasionally a patient (usually a young man) develops severe nodulocystic acne together with a fever, malaise and joint pain and swelling. This is known as acne fulminans.

Pathogenesis of acne

The pathological processes underlying acne remain to be fully elucidated. However, it seems clear that several key features contribute to the final picture. The currently accepted theory is illustrated graphically in Fig. 6.5, but it should be noted that this does not fully explain every aspect of the disorder, for example the occurrence of prepubertal acne.

In essence, the process seems to begin with an increase in sebum production, stimulated by androgens (which are generally in normal amounts even in the most severe cases). At the same time, the mouths of hair follicles with particularly large sebaceous glands, mostly found on the face, neck, chest and back, become blocked by hyperkeratosis. Thus the closed comedo is formed. Within the follicle, an obligate anaerobe *Propionibacterium acnes* proliferates and acts on the sebum, releasing inflammatory chemicals. If these leak into the surrounding dermis, the body mounts an intense acute inflammatory response. The result of this is a papule, pustule or nodule.

As the inflammation subsides, there is a variable tendency to fibrosis. This may produce severe scarring, particularly if repeated episodes occur in the same site. Similarly, large areas may become walled off by fibrosis, leaving cysts.

(a)

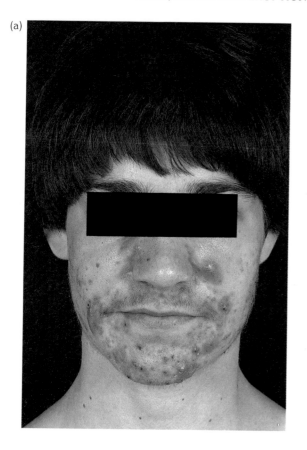

(b)

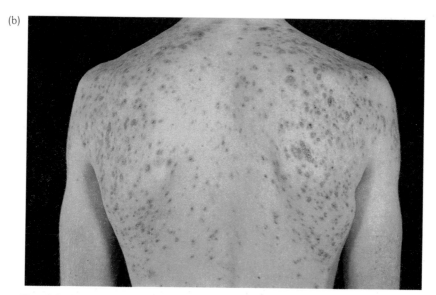

Fig. 6.3. Acne conglobata.

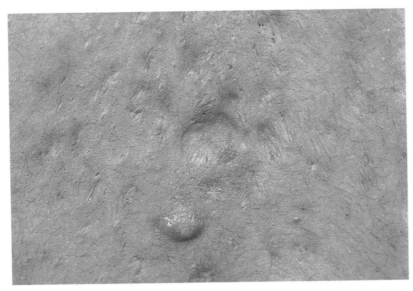

Fig. 6.4. Atrophic scarring in acne.

Treatment of acne

There are a number of useful therapeutic approaches available for the management of acne:

Topical

✗ Benzoyl peroxide 5-10%, gels best
✗ Retinoic acid better desquamator 85-90% cleared,
                                                takes longer
   Sulphur and astringents
   Topical antiseptics
   Topical antibiotics

Systemic
   Antibiotics
   Cyproterone acetate

Accutane 13-cis retinoic acid (isotretinoin) reduces sebum production
   Steroids
   Surgical intervention scar therapy

   mild soap Dove, Dial

Topical therapies

✗ *Benzoyl peroxide* This compound is one of the most widely used anti-acne preparations. Benzoyl peroxide has been shown to reduce the number of comedones (it is 'comedolytic') if used regularly and long term. It also has useful antibacterial activity. It is available in creams, lotions and gels from 2.5% to 10% in strength. It is best to start at the weaker end, applied once daily and gradually increase the strength.

ACNE, ACNEIFORM ERUPTIONS AND ROSACEA   73

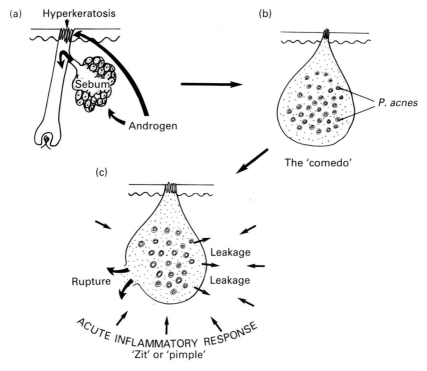

Fig. 6.5. The pathogenesis of acne: (a) At puberty, the surge of circulating androgens stimulates sebum production. Hyperkeratosis also occurs at the mouth of the hair follicle; (b) This results in a dilated chamber, full of sebum, in which an anaerobic organism *Propionibacterium acnes* grows in large numbers: the 'comedo'; and (c) *P. acnes* breaks sebum down into inflammatory chemicals which leak into the surrounding dermis or pour out through a rupture of the follicle wall. This stimulates an intense acute inflammatory infiltrate: the papule or pustule.

✗ *Retinoic acid* This derivative of vitamin A also has comedolytic activity. It is inclined to cause an initial exacerbation in the acne, but is a useful alternative to benzoyl peroxide.

Sulphur and astringents There are a number of preparations which may help to some extent by making the skin surface slightly flaky and thereby unblocking hair follicle orifices.

Topical antiseptics Washes such as povidone iodine and chlorhexidine are often prescribed but are of little proven value in acne.

never use topically   ↙ *best*

Topical antibiotics Tetracycline, erythromycin and clindamycin are all available in topical forms. They are generally used once daily and have all been shown to be useful in milder cases of acne.

Combos – Benzamycin 3% eryth 5% benzoyl perox.

Systemic therapies

③ *Doxycycline* ④ *minocycline*

Antibiotics It is not known exactly how antibiotics work in acne. However, to be effective, they must be fat soluble (*penicillins are therefore of no value at all*). Antibiotics certainly reduce bacterial counts, at least initially, but they may also have direct chemical effects. The tetracyclines in particular are also thought to act by interfering with aspects of the inflammatory process. ①

The most effective oral antibiotics in acne are the tetracycline group and ② erythromycin. Most tetracyclines should be taken on an empty stomach, although this is not so critical for some. There is otherwise little to choose between them. If tetracyclines are contraindicated (for example under the age of 12, in pregnancy or lactation), or if they cannot be tolerated, erythromycin is an excellent substitute. *bacteriostatic, inhibit lipase product. by P. acnes*

abdom cramping? candida vag *inf*

Cyproterone acetate This is an orally effective anti-androgen and can only be given to women. It must be combined with an oestrogen to prevent menorrhagia and to ensure contraceptive cover (it will feminize a male fetus). It has a definite, if slow, effect in acne.

13-cis retinoic acid (isotretinoin) This is a highly effective drug in the management of acne. It is derived from vitamin A and appears to work largely by dramatically reducing sebum production. It has a number of side-effects: dry lips, eyes and skin, nosebleeds, mild alopecia, aches and pains. It also raises blood fat levels and may affect liver function tests. The most serious problem is that it is highly teratogenic so that girls must take adequate contraceptive precautions.

cheilitis conjunctivitis *Pruitis Conjun*

However, over 90% of the patients treated with the drug show complete clearance of their acne and in most there is no relapse. It is available only on hospital prescription in the UK.

Accutane

Steroids These can be used intralesionally or systemically in severe acne.

Surgical intervention Occasionally surgical techniques may be required. Simple measures, such as removing multiple comedones with a comedone extractor may improve the overall appearance. It can certainly give pleasure and satisfaction to a girl- or boyfriend who like to pop out the blackheads. More important, however, is that large, residual cysts may need to be excised. This is generally straightforward, although there is always a risk of keloid scarring. Plastic surgeons can also sometimes help acne scarring by dermabrading the skin, but this must not be attempted until the acne is burnt out or completely under control. *Dermabrasion   acid peels   Zyderm inject.*

Management of a patient with acne

The approach required for each patient should obviously be tailored to the individual, but there are some general guidelines which may be helpful. It is important initially to dispel some myths:

1 Inform the patient that diet plays no role in the production of acne. There is therefore no need to avoid sweets, chocolate or fatty foods.
2 Acne does not arise from a lack of cleanliness.
3 Acne is not usually due to 'hormonal imbalance', nor is it related to sexual behaviour.

In considering specific management further, it is useful to consider acne in three broad severity bands: mild; moderate; and severe.

Mild acne This is acne in which only comedones are present, or in which there are only a few papulopustular lesions, generally restricted to the face.
  Topical treatment alone may control mild acne. It is best to begin with benzoyl peroxide (or retinoic acid), perhaps together with a topical antiseptic or antibiotic preparation as well.

Moderate acne More papulopustular lesions are present on the face or over a wider area. Occasional nodules may occur.
  In general, first-line treatment of moderate acne should combine topical benzoyl peroxide with oxytetracycline or erythromycin in a dose of 500 mg twice daily. This should be continued for at least 3–6 months before considering treatment a failure. Alternative tetracyclines have their advocates. Some may be better absorbed or tolerated, but most are more expensive than oxytetracycline and there is generally no indication for their use as first-line agents.
  If there has not been a satisfactory response to such a regime, the acne should be managed as outlined below for severe acne.

Severe acne It is reasonable to treat acne as severe in four different clinical situations:
1 Largely papulopustular acne but with many, widespread lesions and scarring.
2 Nodulocystic acne.
3 Acne of moderate severity which has failed to settle with 6 months of conventional therapy.
4 Acne of lesser severity which is causing psychological problems.
5 Acne with systemic symptoms (fever, malaise, arthritis: 'acne fulminans').
  Although antibiotic therapy may help to some extent, this degree of acne demands more aggressive treatment. Girls may be treated with cyproterone actetate combined with an oestrogen for a period of at least 6 months. Young men require 13-*cis* retinoic acid. This is given for 4 months at a dose of 1 mg/kg.)
  Intralesional steroids are often useful in suppressing acute inflammatory lesions and very rarely, systemic steroid therapy may be required to control acne fulminans (see above).
  Surgical intervention may be required to help overcome the devastation wreaked by this degree of acne.

Secondary acne
There are several situations in which the lesions of acne may arise as a consequence of other primary pathological processes. Secondary acne is usually rather monomorphic and is generally mild.

Endocrine-associated acne
Typical acne lesions may occur in patients with a number of endocrine abnormalities. The commonest is the polycystic ovary syndrome, in which mild–moderate acne accompanies hirsutism (see Chapter 13) and menstrual irregularities. Any cause of abnormally high circulating androgen levels (such as tumours) may also cause acne, as may Cushing's syndrome.

Medicament-induced acne
The use of greasy ointments and pomades on the skin often induces comedones, particularly on the forehead and cheeks. Occasionally, papules may develop. Topical steroids also induce comedones.
    Several drugs induce acneiform lesions, or make pre-existing acne worse, for example systemic steroids, phenytoin, isoniazid and lithium.

Oil-induced acne
Workers handling mineral oils which come into close contact with the skin often develop acne at unusual sites, such as the lower abdomen and thighs.

Chloracne
Several outbreaks of a systemic upset accompanied by marked comedo formation have resulted from industrial exposure to a variety of chlorinated chemical compounds. A famous example was the release of dioxin from the explosion at Seveso in Italy.

[handwritten annotations: Poral Occlusion Syndrome { H.S. / Acne conglobata / Diss. cellulitis of scalp]

X **Hidradenitis suppurativa**
Hidradenitis suppurativa is a rare but distinctive disorder in which chronic, relapsing sepsis occurs in the apocrine glands of the axillae and groins (Fig. 6.6). Occasionally lesions appear on the breasts (which are modified apocrine glands).
    There are recurrent abscesses and sinus tracks in the affected areas. Comedones also develop. The lesions may be very painful. If severe, the groins and axillae may be replaced by suppurating masses. Many patients with hidradenitis have concurrent bad acne or have suffered with acne in the past. Some patients improve on long-term antibiotics, but many require plastic surgery.

Acneiform disorders
There are several conditions which may mimic acne, but in which close clinical examination will reveal important differences. It is important to distinguish them because treatment is not necessarily the same.

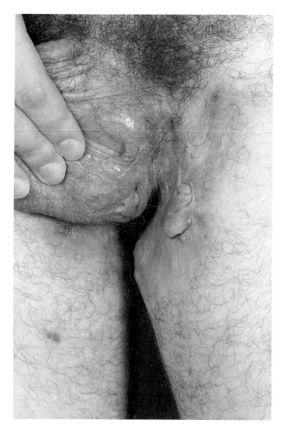

Fig. 6.6. Hidradenitis suppurativa.

Pseudofolliculitis barbae

In this condition, small papules appear in the beard area. It is commoner in those with naturally curly hair, especially Afro-Caribbeans. Occasionally these papules result in small keloids. Similar lesions occasionally develop on the nape of the neck, when it is usually termed *acne keloidalis*. There is no satisfactory treatment.

Acne excoriée (des jeunes filles)

Occasionally a patient (usually a teenage girl) presents with a number of excoriated papules on the face. Careful examination reveals no primary lesions at all. In particular, there are no comedones. This is not true acne but a form of neurotic excoriation (see Chapter 20). Treatment is difficult, but tranquillizers may help.

Pityrosporum folliculitis

Small follicular papules and pustules on the trunk, in the absence of other features of acne, may be due to pityrosporum folliculitis. The condition responds to antifungal agents such as miconazole.

Fig. 6.7. Keratosis pilaris on the upper arm.

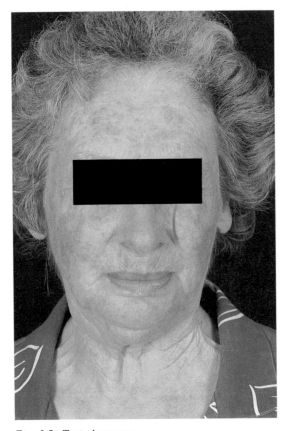

Fig. 6.8. Typical rosacea.

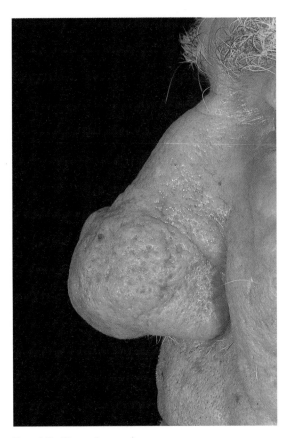

Fig. 6.9. Rhinophyma.

Keratosis pilaris

This is a very common condition in which small spiky projections appear at the mouth of hair follicles. It is frequently hereditary. The commonest sites are the upper outer arms and shoulders, where it is no more than a cosmetic nuisance (Fig. 6.7). However, lesions may appear on the face, especially in children, and may be pustular. Topical retinoic acid may be helpful.

Rosacea

This is an important differential diagnosis of acne, and is sometimes called 'acne rosacea'. It most frequently affects middle-aged woman, but it may certainly occur in men and can occur much earlier in life.

The sites of predilection are the central cheeks, the forehead and glabellar region, the end of the nose and the chin (Fig. 6.8). The eruption characteristically consists of small papules and pustules arising in crops on an erythematous, telangiectatic background. There are no comedones. At a later stage, severe involvement of the nose leads to marked sebaceous hyperplasia: rhinophyma (Fig. 6.9). Patients frequently complain that their face flushes easily in response to heat or alcohol. Migraines are more common.

The treatment of choice is tetracycline antibiotics. These should be given for several weeks in similar doses to those used for moderate acne (see above). Topical sulphur/salicylic acid creams may also help. It may be possible to tail off the treatment in due course, but the condition often recurs. Topical steroids make matters worse.

Peri-oral dermatitis (strict classical scholars would insist on 'circum-oral') produces a clinical appearance somewhat reminiscent of rosacea, and is often associated with topical steroid abuse. This is dealt with in Chapter 22.

Chapter 7
Eczema

To keep three or four spots of eczema in a private part of my
body and now and then to scald or bathe them with hot water
behind closed doors.
Ah, is this not happiness?

(Tim Shangt'an)

The terms eczema and dermatitis are synonymous. They are applied to a
particular type of inflammatory reaction pattern in the skin which may be
provoked by a number of external or internal factors.

Clinical features

The principal symptom of eczema is itching. The changes in the skin seen in
eczema depend on its aetiology, site, and duration, but usually comprise
erythema, oedema, papules, vesicles, and exudation (Fig. 7.1). An acute
eczema will have all these features, and may also have a bullous component. In
a chronic eczema oedema it is not a prominent feature, but the epidermis
becomes thickened and the skin surface markings exaggerated (lichenification).
A common feature of chronic eczema of the hands and feet is the formation of
painful fissures in the skin overlying joints.

A phenomenon which is seen particularly with an acute dermatitis is
secondary spread of the eczema to sites distant from the originally affected area.
In some cases this response is triggered by an external allergen, but in others

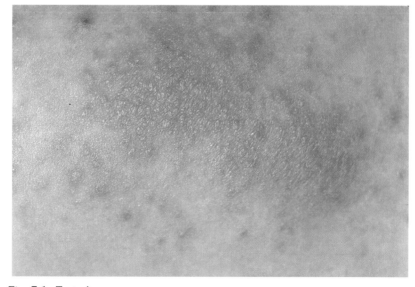

Fig. 7.1. Typical eczema.

there is no obvious explanation for it. Occasionally, most of the body surface is affected, and eczema is one cause of generalized exfoliative dermatitis.

Other changes in the skin which may accompany eczema include scratch marks and secondary bacterial infection. Prolonged scratching and rubbing the skin tends to polish finger-nails, and it is not uncommon to see patients with chronic eczema who look as if they have been using clear nail varnish.

Classification

We still have a great deal to learn about the aetiology of certain types of eczema, so any attempt at classification is based upon our present state of ignorance. The most frequently employed system of classification divides cases of eczema into 'exogenous' where an external agent is responsible, and 'endogenous' where the problem is principally constitutional. There are, however, frequent cases in which more than one factor may be operating—for example the hairdresser with hand dermatitis who suffers from atopic eczema and also has a superimposed irritant dermatitis from shampoos. Don't be too rigid in your attempts to classify a particular dermatitis—it may not fit a recognized category, and you may find yourself using more general terms such as 'probably endogenous'. The following classification includes most of the types of eczema you are likely to encounter:

Exogenous
  Primary irritant dermatitis
  Allergic contact dermatitis
Endogenous
  Atopic eczema
  Seborrhoeic dermatitis
  Discoid eczema
  Varicose eczema
  Endogenous eczema of palms and soles
  Asteatotic eczema

Exogenous eczema

Primary irritant dermatitis

Primary irritants are chemicals which physically damage the skin, and include acids, alkalis, detergents, and petroleum products. Some strong irritants will produce an immediate effect on the skin, whereas with weaker irritants the effects are cumulative. Anyone suffering from a constitutional eczema is more susceptible to the effects of primary irritants because their already abnormal skin has impaired barrier function. The busy housewife with a bone-idle husband, eight children and no washing machine is a good candidate for a cumulative primary irritant dermatitis of the hands, because her hands will be perpetually immersed in washing-up liquid, dirty nappies and soap-powder. However, the wife of a merchant banker with 2.2 children, all mod. cons., a nanny and an au pair, is hardly likely to inconvenience her epidermis to the same degree. The typical appearance of housewives' hand dermatitis is dryness of the palms and finger-tips, sometimes with painful fissures in the skin creases and on the finger pulps.

Occupational irritant dermatitis is a frequent reason for dermatological referral. Hairdressing apprentices are a group who are expected to spend a substantial part of their apprenticeship with their hands immersed in shampoo on their clients' heads, in fact in the early part of their training they do little else. It is hardly surprising that a considerable number develop irritant dermatitis. If they also have a constitutional eczema, such as atopic eczema, their hand problem usually becomes so severe that they are forced to leave hairdressing (Fig. 7.2). A similar situation is seen in machine-tool operators whose hands are immersed in cutting fluids for most of the day.

In theory the treatment of primary irritant dermatitis is simple—either remove the patient from the source of the irritant, or protect the hands against it. This may be feasible in some occupations, but in others it is not. With present employment problems most people are reluctant to give up their jobs, and hairdressers and machine-tool operators usually find it very difficult wearing gloves at work. The skin can be helped to a certain extent by the liberal use of emollients (greasy and oily preparations designed to lubricate the skin), but it cannot be restored to normal whilst exposure to irritants continues. Barrier creams are of no value. What usually happens is that severe dermatitis eventually forces a change of occupation (except in the case of the housewife, who can only consider divorce and aiming for a higher income bracket next time), and individuals with milder problems learn to put up with them.

Allergic contact dermatitis

This is a manifestation of a delayed hypersensitivity reaction to an external allergen. There are innumerable chemicals which can act as allergens, but most

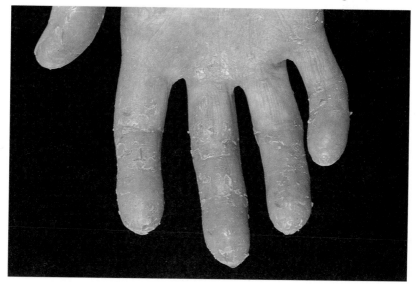

Fig. 7.2. Severe dermatitis of the hands in a hairdresser.

of them rarely cause any problems. Some chemicals are such potent allergens that they will sensitize after one exposure, but many require multiple exposures before sensitization occurs. It is possible to be exposed to a particular allergen for a period of years, and for no apparent reason suddenly develop a hypersensitivity to it.

Frequent causes of contact dermatitis include nickel, colophony, rubber additives, chromate, hair dyes, and topical medicaments—both their active ingredients and preservatives present in their bases.

Nickel dermatitis   Nickel is the commonest cause of contact dermatitis in women. Sensitization to nickel usually occurs in childhood and early adult life as a result of wearing cheap costume jewellery. The problem usually begins with sore, itchy ear-lobes. The advice from female relatives is to discard the cheap earrings and wear good quality gold, or to stop wearing earrings altogether. It is not sore ears which bring the nickel-sensitive girl to the dermatologist, but problems caused by other metallic bits and pieces scattered throughout her accoutrements. In the pre mini-skirt era, suspender dermatitis was the commonest presentation of nickel dermatitis. Suspender belts were perhaps rather more functional than decorative in those days, and the bare metal clips produced patches of dermatitis on the thighs. With the advent of the mini-skirt and the necessity of wearing tights whilst thus attired, suspender dermatitis became a thing of the past. A recent resurgence of interest in the decorative suspender belt has not caused any dermatological problems, because most of the clips are coated metal or synthetic material. It is the humble jeans stud which has become the principal source of nickel on the modern girl. A patch of eczema adjacent to the umbilicus is virtually pathognomonic of nickel sensitivity (Fig. 7.3). If nickel dermatitis is suspected look at the skin under bra clips, wrist-watches and bracelets. Nickel dermatitis on the wrists is usually caused by cheap metal buckles on watch straps, but in women may be due to metal bracelets. Stainless steel in wrist-watches does not appear to cause any problems because although steel contains nickel it is tightly bound and does not leach out.

Any woman who is nickel sensitive should be advised to avoid cheap costume jewellery, bare metal clips in underwear, metal buckles on shoes and metal zips. The metal stud on the front of jeans can be replaced by a button, and problems from watches can usually be avoided by wearing a 'Swatch' watch, as the only metal in contact with the skin is the stainless steel battery compartment.

Colophony   This is a resin which is a component of some adhesive plasters such as Elastoplast.

Rubber dermatitis   Natural latex is a rare sensitizer, but the rubber we encounter in day to day life contains numerous chemicals which can cause contact dermatitis. Several chemicals are used to speed up the vulcanization of rubber (accelerators) and to prevent its oxidation (antioxidants). Rubber glove dermatitis used to be relatively common, but is less frequent nowadays.

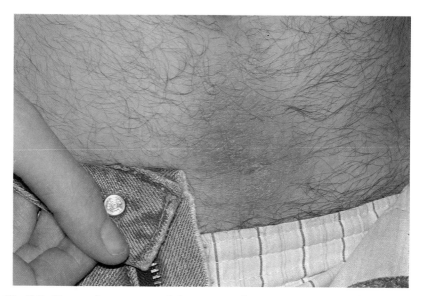

Fig. 7.3. Contact dermatitis to nickel in jeans stud.

Probably the commonest presentation of rubber contact dermatitis is shoe dermatitis—provoked by rubber components and rubber adhesives in shoes.

Chromates   Chromium compounds have a number of industrial applications, they are also used in leather tanning, and they are the major sensitizer in cement. Cement dermatitis is not uncommon in building workers, and has an unfortunate tendency to persist after the patient has been removed from the source of the allergen.

Hair dye dermatitis   Contact dermatitis to a hair dye usually presents with a severe eczema affecting the ears, face and eyelids, as well as scalp involvement. Hair dyes are also frequent causes of allergic contact dermatitis on the hands in hairdressers.

Topical medicaments   Contact dermatitis provoked by topical medicaments is quite common in dermatological practice, but relatively infrequent if one considers the huge quantities of creams, lotions and potions used in an average household. Open any bathroom cabinet or bedside drawer in any house in the land and you will find creams for dry skin, creams for haemorrhoids, preparations for cuts and grazes, creams for insect bites and stings, and almost invariably a tube of topical steroid—originally prescribed for Grandma's varicose eczema, but subsequently used on every cutaneous lesion in sight, including the dog's mange.

Common causes of contact dermatitis in topical medicaments include antibiotics, particularly neomycin, local anaesthetics (except lignocaine which is a rare sensitizer), antihistamines, preservatives such as parabens and ethylenediamine, and lanolin. Dermatoses in which medicament contact sensitivity is a common complicating factor include otitis externa, pruritus ani and varicose ulcers.

Occupational contact dermatitis

If occupational factors are thought to be responsible for contact dermatitis in a patient, a detailed history, including precise information about the nature of the work, is absolutely essential. A history of significant improvement of the dermatitis during holiday periods is typical of a work-related dermatosis. If someone tells you he is a saggar-maker's bottom knocker, enquire as to the precise nature of his colourful employment—it is common to encounter terminology which is specific for certain occupations, and incomprehensible to those outside the trade. Establish what materials are handled at work, and if there have been any recent changes which coincided with the onset of the dermatitis. It is also useful to know if any workmates have similar problems.

A few dermatologists specialize in industrial dermatology, and a great deal of their time is occupied by factory visits. It is frequently essential to see a patient in his working environment to determine what the possible causes of his dermatitis might be.

Plant dermatitis

Allergic contact dermatitis to plants is relatively uncommon in Great Britain but the Primulae, particularly *Primula obconica*, are the plants usually responsible. In the USA the commonest cause of plant dermatitis is poison ivy. Dermatitis caused by plants tends to present with a linear, streaked vesiculobullous reaction on the exposed parts of the body.

Diagnosis of allergic contact dermatitis

It is important to take a detailed history covering present occupation, previous occupations, hobbies, and the use of topical medicaments. In many cases the distribution pattern of the dermatitis will suggest a possible allergen, and provoke further questions—for example, eczema adjacent to the umbilicus prompts questions about previous problems with earrings. Certain patterns are absolutely characteristic of a particular allergen—eczema on the face, in the ears, on the hands, and on one or other thigh is typical of contact sensitivity to phosphorus sesquisulphide in 'strike anywhere' matches. The facial eczema is caused by particles of this chemical in the smoke from the matches; the hand eczema by handling the box, which has the chemical on the striking surface; that on the thigh from carrying the box in the pocket; and that in the ears from using matches to clean them out!

When the cause is not so obvious it may require considerable detective work to track it down. The procedure known as patch testing is of considerable help in the investigation of cases of allergic contact dermatitis. Patch testing is quite different from scratch testing—the former is a delayed hypersensitivity response in which the reaction takes approximately 48 h to develop, whereas the latter is an immediate hypersensitivity response in which a reaction develops within minutes. A standard battery of common allergens is used in routine patch testing, but other batteries of allergens encountered in particular occupations are also available. The majority of the allergens used are mixed with white soft paraffin to a speciffic concentration—many allergens are irritant in high concentration and will produce false positive reactions. Patients will often claim they are 'allergic' to some foul-smelling, highly volatile material they use at work, which is usually presented to the dermatologist in an unmarked jar. These unknown materials are often irritants and if used undiluted for patch testing will probably bore a large, untidy hole in the patient's back.

A small quantity of each patch test agent is applied to filter paper discs on aluminium strips (A1-test tape), or aluminium chambers on Scanpore tape (Finn chambers) and these are placed in rows on the patient's back. The strips are numbered so that each agent can be identified. The patch tests are removed after 48 h, and a positive reaction is indicated by a small area of eczema (Fig. 7.4). The back is then examined after a further interval of 48 h to detect any late reactions. Positive reactions must be interpreted in the context of the patient's presenting problem—not all positives will be relevant.

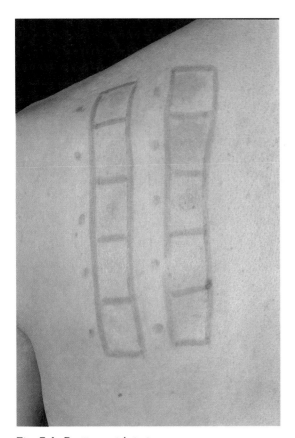

Fig. 7.4. Positive patch tests.

Wait until an acute eczema has settled before patch testing—positive reactions may exacerbate the eczema.

Treatment

Potent topical steroids (see Chapter 22) should be used to settle the eczema prior to patch testing. Once an allergen has been identified as the cause of the problem, the patient should be given advice about its avoidance—typed information sheets are useful for this. If components of medicaments are involved, the patient's general practitioner should be informed of what preparations to avoid in future.

Endogenous eczema

Atopic eczema

Atopy is a term applied to a common genetic predisposition to develop eczema, asthma and hay fever. A family history of atopy is found in the majority of patients suffering from atopic eczema. The pathogenesis of atopic eczema is complex, and in addition to a constitutional predisposition other factors such as environmental influences, and emotional stimuli may contribute to the problem.

Atopic eczema is not present at birth, but frequently appears within the first year of life, often between the ages of 2 and 4 months. In early childhood the eczema is often generalized, but in older children a characteristic pattern of involvement of limb flexures is seen—wrists, antecubital fossae, popliteal fossae, and dorsa of feet (Fig. 7.5). The typical picture in older children and adults is of facial eczema, hand eczema, flexural eczema on the limbs, and some involvement of the trunk. The skin is extremely dry, and intensely itchy. In time,

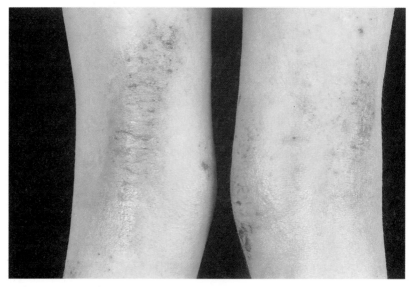

Fig. 7.5. Flexural involvement in atopic eczema.

as a result of constant scratching and rubbing, affected areas of skin become thickened (lichenification). The course of atopic eczema is typically punctuated by episodic exacerbations.

In many, atopic eczema will resolve in childhood, but in others it persists into adolescence and adult life. There is no certain way of predicting the outcome in an individual. Those whose eczema has cleared remain particularly susceptible to the effects of primary irritants on the skin. They should avoid occupations such as hairdressing and engineering in which the hands are frequently exposed to primary irritants.

The commonest complication of atopic eczema is secondary bacterial infection, producing folliculitis or impetigo. Viral warts and molluscum contagiosum occur more frequently in atopics, and herpes simplex infection may lead to widespread skin lesions (see Chapter 3) and a severe illness (eczema herpeticum; Kaposi's varicelliform eruption).

Treatment

The most important aspect of the management of a child with atopic eczema is sympathetic explanation of the nature of the condition to its parents.

Emollients are designed to moisturize the skin, and are essential in the management of the dry skin in atopic eczema. There are numerous proprietary emollients available, and it may be necessary to swap and change preparations to find those most suitable for a particular individual. They can be used in combination at bathtime—for example, emulsifying ointment as a soap substitute, a bath oil (Oilatum emollient; Alpha Keri bath oil; Balneum) in the water, and an emollient cream (Boots E45 cream; Oilatum cream; Unguentum Merck) after bathing.

Topical steroids are invaluable in the treatment of atopic eczema. They are available in a variety of strengths (see Chapter 22). In young children mild, non-fluorinated steroids such as hydrocortisone are the mainstay of topical therapy. In older children and adults more potent steroids are required, but the aim should always be to use the weakest preparation sufficient to control the disease. A topical steroid/antibacterial combination may be useful in individuals whose eczema frequently becomes secondarily infected—obvious secondary infection should be treated with a systemic antibiotic such as flucloxacillin or erythromycin.

Medicated bandages such as Ichthopaste and Coltapaste are useful in the management of severe eczema on the limbs. The bandages may be applied over a topical steroid, and changed every 2 or 3 days. A sedative antihistamine at night may help to reduce scratching, but often it would seem to be more beneficial to prescribe it for the parents. Ultraviolet light treatment helps some atopics, but unfortunately the eczema relapses quite rapidly when treatment is stopped.

The influence of diet on atopic eczema is a rather contentious matter. In some children, replacement of cows' milk by a soya preparation results in some improvement in the eczema, but in the majority it does not appear to help. Most dermatologists reserve dietary manipulation for those severely affected children who have obtained no benefit from other treatment methods. It is potentially dangerous to manipulate a child's diet without expert advice, as this can lead to nutritional deficiencies.

Seborrhoeic dermatitis

This is a constitutional disorder whose exact pathogenesis is not fully understood. Recently, the role of Pityrosporum yeasts in its provocation has been emphasized.

Seborrhoeic dermatitis may affect the scalp, face, presternal area, upper back, and flexures. Scalp involvement presents as itchy, diffuse scaling on an erythematous background. Seborrhoeic dermatitis on the face typically produces scaly erythema in the nasolabial folds, but may be more extensive and involve the forehead, eyebrows, beard area and ears (Fig. 7.6). On the presternal area the lesions are often marginated. Flexural involvement produces a moist, glazed erythema.

Seborrhoeic dermatitis usually responds to treatment with topical hydrocortisone preparations, but will recur when treatment is stopped. It is important to explain this to the patient, who will otherwise be tempted to try more and

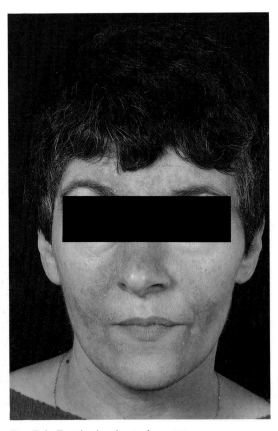

Fig. 7.6. Facial seborrhoeic dermatitis.

more potent topical steroids in an attempt to find a 'cure'. Tar shampoos and topical steroid lotions or gels will help the scalp problem. The apparent involvement of Pityrosporum in the pathogenesis of this condition has prompted the use of topical ketoconazole (Nizoral) cream, and more recently a shampoo preparation, both of which appear to be beneficial.

Discoid eczema

In this pattern of eczema scattered, well-demarcated areas are present on the trunk and limbs. A potent topical steroid is usually required to keep the condition controlled. Its aetiology is unknown.

Varicose (stasis: gravitational) eczema

Chronic venous stasis is frequently associated with eczematous changes on the legs. Itchy areas of eczema develop in association with haemosiderin pigmentation. Secondary spread to the forearms is common.

Mild or moderate potency topical steroids will usually help suppress the eczema.

Endogenous eczema of palms and soles

Some patients develop a symmetrical pattern of eczema affecting the palms and soles which is chronic, and does not appear to be related to any external factors. Treatment usually involves long-term potent topical steroid therapy.

An episodic form of eczema of the palms and soles in which bulla formation occurs is known as *acute pompholyx* (Fig. 7.7). This develops rapidly, and can be severely incapacitating. Secondary bacterial infection is common. It usually

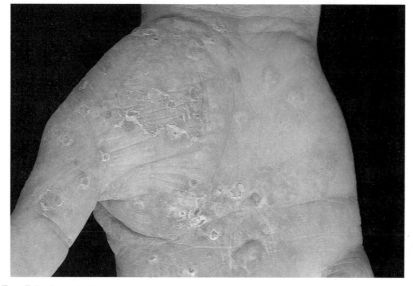

Fig. 7.7. Pompholyx.

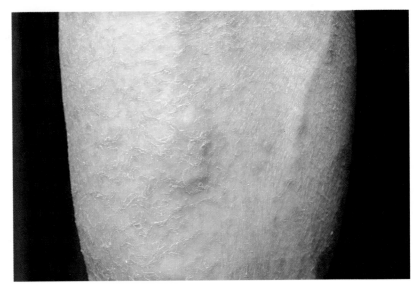

Fig. 7.8. Eczema craquelé.

responds well to treatment with potassium permanganate soaks and a systemic antibiotic. The trigger for these acute episodes is unknown.

Asteatotic eczema (eczema craquelé)

With increasing age, the lipid content of the stratum corneum decreases, and the elderly skin is particularly susceptible to drying and 'degreasing' agents. Asteatotic eczema is usually seen on the legs, but may also occur on the lower abdomen and arms, and occasionally it is generalized. It is a common problem in elderly patients admitted to hospital, particularly for surgical procedures, and bathed rather more frequently than they bathe at home. The dry stratum corneum cracks into a crazy-paving pattern (Fig. 7.8), and the skin begins to itch. Treatment with an emollient at this stage is usually sufficient, but if not treated, a more troublesome exudative eczema often develops, and this will require topical steroid therapy.

Chapter 8
Psoriasis

Psoriasis is one of the commonest and most important of the inflammatory dermatoses. It has been estimated that about 1.5% of the population of most Western countries can expect to suffer from psoriasis during their lifetime and it is also common in India, the Far East, and parts of Africa. As most of those who develop psoriasis are stuck with it in some form or other for the rest of their lives, it is clearly a considerable problem.

It is still not precisely known why some people develop psoriasis. It seems that there is a strong genetic component in some, particularly those in whom the disease begins in youth or early adulthood. However, although a family history is common, there is often no clear-cut inheritance pattern and the 'genetic' explanation may not be readily understood by many patients.

There are some well-recognized triggers which may induce psoriasis in susceptible individuals, such as trauma and infections. Some authorities believe that stress may also induce or exacerbate psoriasis. However, there is no clear understanding of what it is that causes some areas of skin to turn into plaques of psoriasis while others remain essentially normal. A great deal of research has been, and is being, devoted to trying to answer this question. Although a number of biochemical and other abnormalities have been demonstrated, it is not known whether these are primary defects or secondary to the disease process.

The underlying pathological process is a combination of disturbed hyper-proliferation of the epidermis accompanied by accumulations of inflammatory cells. The epidermal transit time is markedly reduced from the normal 30 days to around 6 days. There is also increased vascularity of the upper dermis. Fig. 8.1 shows a schematic representation of a psoriatic plaque. The cardinal features are:

1 Marked thickening of the epidermis: acanthosis.
2 Absence of the granular cell layer.
3 Retention of nuclei in the horny layer: parakeratosis.
4 Accumulations of polymorphs in the horny layer: microabscesses.
5 Dilated capillary loops in the upper dermis.

This basic pathological picture with some variations (e.g. increased size and number of polymorph abscesses in pustular psoriasis) unites all forms of psoriasis. It is also seen in the skin lesions that may accompany Reiter's syndrome (see below).

Clinical patterns

A number of different clinical patterns of psoriasis are recognized:
    Classical plaque

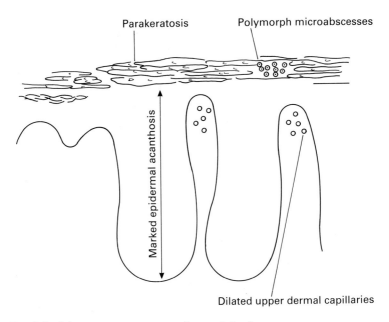

Parakeratosis   Polymorph microabscesses

Marked epidermal acanthosis

Dilated upper dermal capillaries

Fig. 8.1. Schematic representation of a psoriatic plaque.

Scalp psoriasis
Nail psoriasis
Guttate
Flexural
'Brittle'
Erythrodermic
Acute pustular
Chronic palmoplantar pustulosis
Arthropathic psoriasis

Some are common and some are rarer and some may be seen together or overlapping with each other. However, there is some merit in considering them separately. We shall deal first with the so-called 'classical' or plaque form of the condition, and also with scalp, nail and joint changes, before covering the other patterns of psoriatic skin involvement.

Classical plaque psoriasis

This is the commonest pattern. There are single or multiple plaques, varying from a few millimetres to several centimetres across. The plaques are red, and the surface is scaly (Fig. 8.2). If scraped very gently, the scale can be seen to reflect the light, giving a 'silvery' effect. This is due to the parakeratotic horny layer. More vigorous rubbing of the plaque induces capillary point haemorrhage.

The plaques may be anywhere on the body surface but psoriasis has a predilection for the extensor surfaces: the knees, the elbows and the base of the spine. The lesions are often strikingly symmetrical. Involvement of the face is

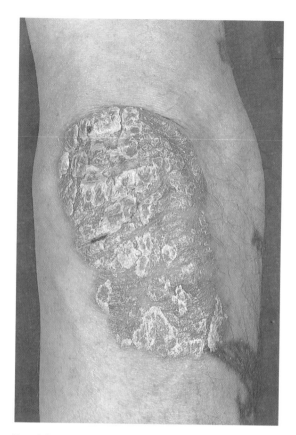

Fig. 8.2. Psoriatic plaque on the elbow.

relatively uncommon. The scalp and nails are often affected and an arthropathy may also occur (see below).

The lesions tend to be very chronic and stable, with little day to day change (as compared to 'brittle' psoriasis—see below). However, plaques do grow slowly and may merge with adjacent plaques. They also disappear from time to time. Occasionally, psoriatic plaques may appear at the site of trauma or scarring. This is known as the Köbner or isomorphic phenomenon and is a characteristic, but not pathognomonic, feature of psoriasis. Conversely, exposure to UV radiation and natural sunlight often (but not always) improve psoriasis.

It is often said that psoriasis is not itchy, but it is our experience that a significant minority of patients complain of quite severe itching and that most patients experience some itch at times. In fact the Greek 'psora', from which the name is derived, actually means itch. Some forms of psoriasis (e.g. guttate, flexural) are more prone to cause irritation than chronic plaque psoriasis.

There are no consistent laboratory abnormalities in patients with psoriasis, but some have a raised serum uric acid level.

Scalp psoriasis

Scalp involvement in psoriasis is very common. Indeed the scalp may be the only affected area. It is sometimes difficult to distinguish scalp psoriasis from bad seborrhoeic dermatitis (see also flexural psoriasis below), but psoriasis is generally thicker. It has been said, with some truth, that if scalp lesions can be felt as well as seen, then psoriasis is the likely diagnosis.

Lesions vary in extent from one or two plaques to a sheet of thick scale covering the whole scalp surface (Fig. 8.3). This is shed regularly, leading to severe 'dandruff'. Rarely, the scale becomes very thick indeed and sticks in large chunks to bundles of hair. This is known as 'pityriasis amiantacea'. There may be temporary hair loss in severe scalp psoriasis.

Nail psoriasis

Nail abnormalities are frequently seen in psoriasis. They are, in fact, one of the most useful diagnostic clues if the skin lesions are few and far between or atypical. Nail changes are almost always present in arthropathic psoriasis.

There are two common findings: pitting and onycholysis. Psoriatic nail pits are relatively large and irregularly arranged (Fig. 8.4), as compared with those

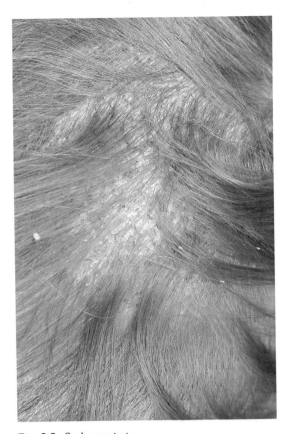

Fig. 8.3. Scalp psoriasis.

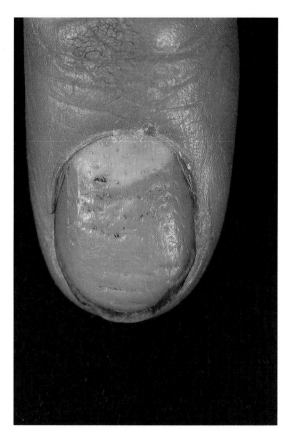

Fig. 8.4. Nail pits in psoriasis.

seen in alopecia areata. Onycholysis (lifting of the nail plate) may accompany pitting or occur separately. It is sometimes painful. When onycholysis is recent, there is a dull area under the nail, with a salmon pink rim (Fig. 8.5). Later the nail often becomes discoloured brown or yellow.

These nail changes, particularly onycholysis, may also occur without other evidence of the disease and some authorities would classify this as isolated nail psoriasis.

In severe psoriasis, such as erythrodermic or pustular forms, more gross nail changes occur. The whole nail surface may become roughened and discoloured. Occasionally, pustular changes occur at the ends of the digits and in the nail bed itself. This is sometimes known as 'acrodermatitis continua'. Similar changes may accompany chronic palmoplantar pustulosis (see below).

Guttate psoriasis

'Gutta' is the Latin for 'drop' and some learned ancient presumably thought that the lesions that cover the patient with 'guttate' psoriasis were intensely drop-like. Most are about about 1 cm in diameter (Fig. 8.6). Guttate psoriasis may be itchy. The colour is usually paler pink than established plaque psoriasis,

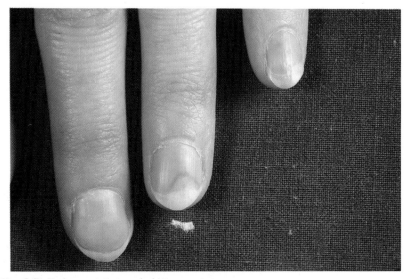

Fig. 8.5. Early psoriatic onycholysis.

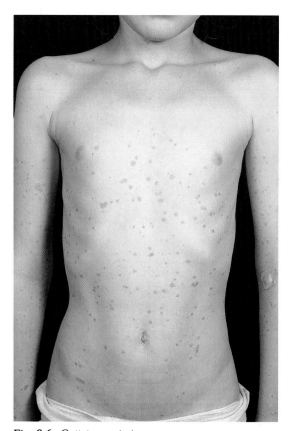

Fig. 8.6. Guttate psoriasis.

at least initially. The main differential diagnosis is pityriasis rosea (*see* Chapter 15). These can best be distinguished by the presence of parakeratotic scale in psoriasis, and the shape of the lesions, which are round in guttate psoriasis and oval in pityriasis rosea.

The guttate form of psoriasis often erupts suddenly and may follow an infection, especially a streptococcal sore throat. It may also disappear rapidly, but in some patients the patches enlarge and become stable plaques.

Flexural psoriasis

Flexural involvement in psoriasis may accompany otherwise typical plaque lesions elsewhere, but it is also quite commonly seen alone, or just with scalp and nail changes. Lesions may occur in any or all of: the groin, natal cleft, axillae, umbilicus and submammary folds. Because of the maceration and friction that inevitably occur in these areas, the surface scale is often lost, leaving a rather beefy erythematous rash (Fig. 8.7). It may be very difficult to distinguish this from flexural seborrhoeic dermatitis if there are no nail changes or evidence of psoriasis elsewhere. Some authorities consider that there is an overlap between these two conditions, and call such changes *sebo-psoriasis*.

Flexural psoriasis is often itchy. The use of proprietary anti-itch preparations may give rise to a secondary contact sensitivity, thus further obscuring the clinical picture.

Brittle psoriasis

Occasionally a patient is encountered whose psoriasis does not consist of thick, stable plaques, but of thin, irritable scaly areas (Fig. 8.8). This type of lesion may develop suddenly in a patient whose psoriasis has been stable for years, or

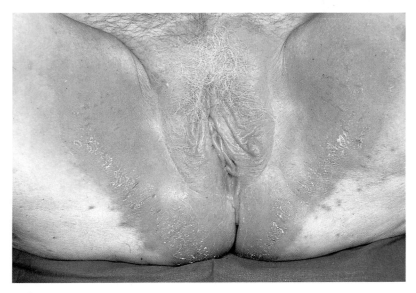

Fig. 8.7. Flexural psoriasis.

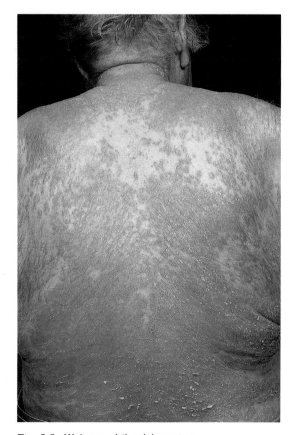

Fig. 8.8. Widespread 'brittle' psoriasis.

it may arise *de novo* as the first type of psoriasis seen in that patient. Such a change may follow systemic steroid therapy (often for another condition), but widespread use of potent topical steroids may also induce stable psoriasis to go 'brittle'.

The significance of brittle psoriasis is that the lesions may rapidly generalize, especially if treated with potent agents (*see* treatment section below), leading to erythroderma or even acute pustular psoriasis.

Erythrodermic psoriasis

When psoriatic plaques merge to cover most, if not the whole, skin surface a state of erythroderma or exfoliative dermatitis results. The effects of this state are covered in Chapter 15.

Psoriasis may become erythrodermic by slow, inexorable progression of the disease, or it may develop rapidly. Occasionally, erythrodermic psoriasis may appear *de novo*. Systemic steroids or the use of potent topical steroid may precipitate this form of the disease.

Acute pustular psoriasis (of von Zumbusch)

This is a very serious form of psoriasis. Patients with or without pre-existing psoriatic lesions suddenly develop widespread areas of erythema. Superimposed on these areas are pustules which may merge and coalesce into lakes of pus (Fig. 8.9). Swabs are sterile.

The patient usually has a high, swinging fever and is toxic and unwell. There is a leucocytosis. If the disease is unchecked, patients become increasingly ill and may die, often of secondary infections.

Chronic palmoplantar pustulosis (pustular psoriasis of palms and soles)

There is some debate as to the precise relationship between this condition and other forms of psoriasis. Although biopsies reveal a distinctly psoriasiform pathology, it is unusual for patients to have chronic palmoplantar pustulosis in association with other types of psoriatic lesion.

The typical changes in palmoplantar pustulosis consist of erythematous patches on the surface of which develop numerous pustules (Fig. 8.10). These pustules gradually change into circular, brown, scaly spots which eventually peel off. The condition is usually uncomfortable or painful, rather than itchy.

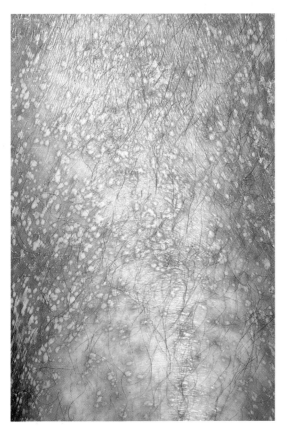

Psoriatic arthritis

≈ R.A. but asymmetr.

7% psor. pt also have jt involvem't

⊖ R.F.

↑ HLA B-27

Fig. 8.9. Acute pustular psoriasis.

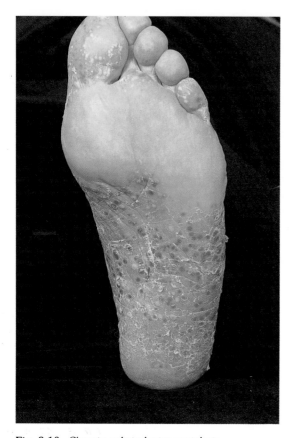

Fig. 8.10. Chronic palmoplantar pustulosis.

Lesions may vary from a small area affecting one hand or foot, to involvement of the entire surface of both palms and soles. This may lead to considerable disability. There may be a nail dystrophy if the lesions extend down a digit.

Treatment

The agents most widely used in the treatment of the skin lesions of psoriasis are:

Topical

Emollients   *Anthalin + UVB*

× Tar   *+ UVB*

Salicylic acid

× Topical steroids

Dithranol (anthralin)

× UV radiation   *UVA, UVB*

Systemic

× PUVA (psoralen + UVA)

Retinoids

× Cytotoxics, e.g. methotrexate

Tegison

Azathioprine
Hydroxyurea
Systemic steroids
Cyclosporin A

It is an old adage that if there are many treatments for a disease, none of them works perfectly. This is true of psoriasis. Although each of the modalities are useful in some patients, none are universally effective and some have a high rate of unwanted effects.

We shall outline each of the modalities in turn and then discuss briefly how these may be used in the major clinical forms of psoriasis.

Topical therapies

There are a number of agents that can be used topically to induce a remission or an improvement in psoriatic skin lesions. Most have the advantage of being entirely safe, but it is not always easy to persuade patients to continue to use topical agents for weeks, months or even years on end.

Emollients

One of the major complaints in psoriasis is the scaling. Some patients are prepared to put up with the presence of the plaques (especially if they are mostly on covered sites) if the scaling can be controlled. Emollients such as white or yellow soft paraffin or lanolin may accomplish this.

Tar

Tar has been used for psoriasis for many years, particularly in combination with UV radiation. The most effective tar preparations are extracts of crude coal tar, often in the form of alcoholic solutions such as liquor picis carbonis. Although attempts have been made to refine tar to make it more cosmetically acceptable, the most effective tar preparations still seem to be those which are the darkest, smelliest and messiest. Consequently, not many patients are prepared to use tar for widespread, routine use. However, tar in bathing emollient oils or in ointment mixtures may be helpful for skin lesions and there is still an important role for tar in treating scalp disease.

Salicylic acid

Salicylic acid is a 'keratolytic' agent and helps to reduce the scaling in psoriatic plaques. It can be used with tar in mixtures, and is also combined with a potent topical steroid in a commercially available preparation.

Topical steroids

Topical steroids do not eradicate psoriatic lesions, but may suppress them temporarily. Some dermatologists never use topical steroids in psoriasis because of the risks of side-effects and of turning the psoriasis 'brittle' (see above). However, if used with care in stable disease, on the scalp and in the flexures, they can be useful.

Dithranol (anthralin)

Dithranol is probably the single most effective topical antipsoriatic treatment. Application of creams and pastes containing dithranol can convert a patch of psoriasis into completely normal-looking skin. The agent is an anthracene derivative and its mode of action is unknown. It has been used in combination with tar and UV radiation for many years (the Ingram regime), and patients can be cleared in about 3 weeks of daily treatment. Originally, dithranol was left in contact with the skin for 24 h, but it is now known that is unnecessary, as half-hour 'short-contact' therapy is just as good.

The most effective preparation is dithranol in Lassar's paste (a mixture of starch, zinc oxide and salicylic acid in white soft paraffin), but dithranol is also commercially available in cream and ointment bases. It is usual to begin with a low concentration (0.1%) and gradually increase this as necessary.

The main complications of dithranol therapy are staining and burning. The staining is due to oxidation of the dithranol to a purplish brown dye. This is temporary on the skin (it peels off with the shed horny cells) but is permanent on baths, bedding and clothes. Dithranol burns can be very unpleasant, especially around the eyes. Patients must therefore be taught how to use dithranol by an experienced doctor or nurse before being advised to use it on their psoriasis.

UV radiation

The use of UV in the treatment of psoriasis is well-established. As already mentioned, exposure to natural sunlight often improves psoriasis. The most effective wavelengths lie in the medium (UVB) range. This requires careful handling, because it is also the part of the UV spectrum that induces sunburn. Patients require doses which just induce erythema but do not cause burning. The dose needs to be increased gradually as the patient develops a tan. Treatment is usually given twice or three times weekly until clearance is achieved. Adjunctive tar may make the UV more effective.

UVB is also carcinogenic (as is tar), but there are surprisingly few psoriatics who develop therapeutically-induced skin cancers from tar or standard UVB.

Systemic therapies

Psoralen + UVA (PUVA)

Psoralens are a group of compounds that form chemical bonds with DNA in the presence of UV radiation. This inhibits DNA replication. The most widely used agent in the treatment of psoriasis is 8-methoxypsoralen, which is usually taken by mouth 2 h before exposure to long-wave UV light (UVA). The patient has to wear protective glasses because of potential ocular damage. Unlike standard UVB, there appears to be a significant risk of keratoses and epithelial cancers in psoriatics treated with PUVA.

Cytotoxic drugs

By far the most effective and widely used of these agents is methotrexate, a folic acid antagonist. This is effective in most cases of psoriasis in a once weekly dosage of between 7.5 and 20 mg.) Other drugs that are sometimes given include azathioprine (which may be especially helpful in arthropathic psoriasis) and hydroxyurea.

All cytotoxics are complicated by unwanted side-effects, particularly bone marrow suppression. Methotrexate only occasionally induces marrow failure in conventional anti-psoriatic doses, but may do so in an idiosynchratic, non-dose-related manner. The major problem with methotrexate is hepatoxicity. This may be acute but this is rare. However, some patients develop later, more insidious changes in the liver, leading ultimately to hepatic fibrosis. Alcohol appears to exacerbate this tendency. There are no reliable non-invasive techniques for assessing this and young patients on methotrexate require annual or biennial liver biopsies. Methotrexate also inhibits spermatogenesis and is teratogenic. These complications restrict its use to severely affected patients for whom there is no alternative.

Retinoids

A new class of vitamin A derivatives has been found to help some patients with psoriasis. The most commonly used at present is etretinate. The effects are unpredictable but may be very rewarding. Retinoids have a number of cutaneous side-effects, including dry lips, nose-bleeds and hair loss. They may also induce a hyperlipidaemia, raise liver enzymes and are teratogenic.

Systemic steroids

In very severe psoriasis, steroids may occasionally be necessary. However, there are usually major difficulties in weaning patients off them, once started, and systemic steroids should be avoided if at all possible.

Cyclosporin A

This very expensive drug has recently been found to work in bad psoriasis. It is nephrotoxic and is still under evaluation.

Treatment of clinical patterns

Chronic plaque psoriasis

Dithranol is ideal for this type of disease. If the patient's life-style, or burning make dithranol impossible, topical steroids, with or without tar and salicylic acid can be used. Ultraviolet radiation is also useful. Some patients will settle for emollients only, if they are not desperate to clear the skin completely.

If lesions become very extensive or if the psoriasis is having serious psychological effects, PUVA, retinoids or cytotoxic drugs may be needed. This decision is a difficult one and depends on each individual patient's specific circumstances.

Scalp psoriasis

Tar shampoos are very helpful in scalp disease, but will seldom control thick plaques on their own. Tar gels may help. A very effective topical remedy is

Unguentum Cocois Co. which is a mixture of, amongst other things, tar and salicylic acid. This is massaged into the scalp at night and washed out the following morning. Topical steroid lotions, with or without salicylic acid are also used.

Nail psoriasis

Nail changes will not respond to topical treatment and systemic drugs are seldom justified for the nails alone.

Guttate psoriasis

This form of psoriasis is most easily treated with UV radiation together with a mild tar-based ointment.

Flexural psoriasis

Psoriasis in the flexures poses considerable management problems. Some patients respond to mild tar–corticosteroid mixtures, but long-term use of topical steroids in the flexures can cause striae. Dithranol, if used in very low concentrations can be managed successfully, but burning is common and underclothes often get stained. Ultraviolet and PUVA generally fail to reach the affected areas.

Brittle psoriasis

Brittle psoriasis needs very gentle management. Potent topical steroids, strong tar and salicylic acid preparations should be withdrawn. Emollients, such as white soft paraffin should be applied twice daily initially until the skin appears to be returning to a more stable condition. If this does not happen, or if the skin deteriorates, PUVA, retinoids or methotrexate should be considered, at least for a short time.

Erythrodermic and acute pustular psoriasis

Although both of these states may settle with conservative management similar to that outlined for brittle psoriasis, it is more likely that they will require systemic treament from the beginning. Such intervention can be life-saving. The most effective agent is methotrexate, used in small doses parenterally twice weekly. When the psoriasis is stabilizing, a single oral weekly dose should be substituted. Later, PUVA and/or retinoids may be added and the cytotoxic gradually reduced or withdrawn. Some patients, however, relapse and require methotrexate long-term.

Chronic palmoplantar pustulosis

Nothing is really effective in this condition. Tar pastes, potent topical steroids or dithranol may work, but they often do not. Oral tetracyclines have their advocates. Psoralen and ultraviolet A to the hands and feet seems to be the best of a bad lot and may control the disease, but it invariably relapses if treatment is stopped.

Arthropathic psoriasis
One of the most unpleasant and difficult complications of psoriasis is the arthropathy that may occur in up to 10% of psoriatics. There are four basic patterns:
1   Distal interphalangeal joint involvement.
2   Seronegative rheumatoid-like joint changes.
3   Large joint mono or polyarthropathy.
4   Spondylitis.

The commonest type of arthropathy seen in psoriatics is that involving the distal interphalangeal joints, with the others listed above in descending order of frequency. Psoriatic arthropathy is erosive and may result in destruction of the joints if severe and unchecked. Psoriatics who develop the spondylitic form are usually HLA B27 positive, and there is a degree of overlap between psoriatic arthropathy and the other triggers of seronegative arthritis such as inflammatory bowel disease and Reiter's syndrome (see below and Chapter 19).

The treatment of arthropathic psoriasis involves the judicious use of drugs known to be useful in the arthritides, such as non-steroidal anti-inflammatory

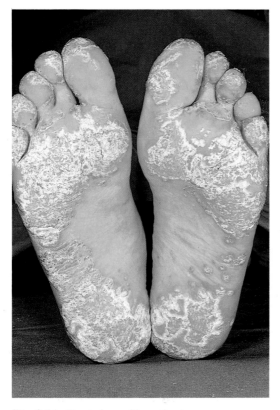

Fig. 8.11. Keratoderma blenorrhagica.

drugs and gold. However, psoriatic arthritis may also respond to systemic anti-psoriatic drugs (see above), especially azathioprine and the retinoids.

Reiter's syndrome

This disorder, which frequently follows a diarrhoeal illness or non-specific urethritis in HLA B27 positive individuals, is discussed in Chapter 19. Occasionally skin lesions known as 'keratoderma blenorrhagica' develop. Palmar and plantar lesions may become very gross (Fig. 8.11), while lesions elsewhere are clinically very similar to psoriasis. Histologically keratoderma blenorrhagica is indistinguishable from psoriasis.

Chapter 9
Benign and Malignant Skin Tumours

Classification of skin tumours

Lumps on or in the skin are common. For example, in our outpatients 27% of the patients have one of nine common types of skin tumour, with a further 19% having viral warts (see Chapter 3). Furthermore, this workload is rising, partly because of the rising age of the population as a whole (many skin tumours are commoner in the elderly) and partly because skin cancer is on the increase in all age groups. Although most skin tumours are benign and often represent only a cosmetic nuisance, it is clearly important to be able to distinguish between these and those which are malignant or of malignant potential. A decision about what can or should be done about any individual lesion can only be made after a diagnosis to this minimum level has been made.

The skin is a complex organ system and there are both benign and malignant tumours described for each and every component. Table 9.1 gives some idea of the wide variety of skin tumours that can occur, although even this is much simplified!

We shall discuss benign tumours first concentrating on the commonest and most important, and then discuss malignant tumours separately. However, some of those which are not specifically mentioned in the text will obviously also be encountered occasionally.

Some skin lumps are hamartomatous malformations due to aberrant development. Such a lesion in the skin is generally termed a 'naevus'. Naevi are discussed separately in Chapter 10.

General treatment principles

It is worth reviewing briefly the techniques that are available for dealing with skin tumours. This will avoid repetition.

The first important principle is that if there is any diagnostic doubt, some tissue should be preserved for histology. Failure to do this will mean missed melanomas and other malignancies and is one of the causes of patients presenting with mysterious lymphatic or distant deposits from unknown cutaneous primary sites.

Surgical removal or biopsy

The technique of biopsy has already been described and illustrated in Chapter 2 (Figs. 2.1, 2.2, 2.3). Removal of small skin tumours under local anaesthetic is quick, simple and cheap. If the tumour is too large for primary excision, a small incisional biopsy should be performed. This should cross the edge from normal to abnormal tissue. There is very little evidence that a biopsy of this kind

Table 9.1. Types of skin tumour

Epidermis (for naevi *see* Chapter 10)
Benign
    Seborrhoeic keratosis
    Skin tags
    Keratoacanthoma
    Clear cell acanthoma
    (viral warts) (*see* Chapter 3)
    Tumours of skin appendages, e.g. sweat glands, sebaceous glands, hair follicles
    Epidermal cysts

Dysplastic/malignant
    Actinic (solar) keratosis
    Squamous cell carinoma
        In situ (Bowen's disease)
        Invasive
    Paget's disease
    Tumours of skin appendages
    Basal cell carcinoma

Melanocytes (for naevi *see* Chapter 10)
Benign
    Freckle and lentigo

Dysplastic/malignant
    Dysplastic naevus (*see* Chapter 10)
    Lentigo maligna
    Malignant melanoma
        Lentigo maligna melanoma
        Superficial spreading
        Nodular
        Acral

Dermis (for naevi *see* Chapter 10)
Benign
    Fibrous tissue
        Dermatofibroma
    Neural tissue
        e.g. neurofibroma
    Vascular tumours
        Angioma/angiokeratoma
        Pyogenic granuloma
        Glomus tumour

Dysplastic/Malignant
    Fibrosarcoma
    Neurofibrosarcoma
    Angiosarcoma including Kaposi's sarcoma

Pseudotumours
    (e.g. chondrodermatitis nodularis helicis; hypertrophic and keloid scars)

Lymphomas
Cutaneous T cell lymphoma (mycosis fungoides)
    B cell lymphoma

Extension from deeper tissues and *metastatic deposits*

---

adversely affects the outcome, although most would try to avoid incisional biopsy of invasive melanomas (see below).

Curettage and/or cautery
This is a perfectly satisfactory method of dealing with superficial tumours. After infiltration of the skin with anaesthetic, a curette (Volkmann spoon) is used to scrape off the lesion. This leaves a raw, oozing base for which a few touches with a simple cautery is usually sufficient. Pedunculated skin tumours can be removed simply by using the cautery across the narrow base. An alternative to cautery is a hyfrecator—a machine which produces electrical haemostasis and dessication.

Cryotherapy
The use of cold in the treatment of tumours has become very popular. It is ideal for superficial skin tumours because it is quick and leaves relatively little scarring. However, histological interpretation of cryobiopsies is not always easy and its use is generally restricted to benign tumours or tumours in which an incisional biopsy has already been performed. Cryotherapy is not appropriate for melanomas other than lentigo maligna (see below).

The best substance to use is liquid nitrogen which may be applied with cotton wool on a stick, or by spray or probe using specially designed instruments. The lesion is frozen until a halo of frozen skin 1 mm around the tumour is obtained. This should be maintained for 10 s for benign lesions and 30 s for malignant tumours. This should be allowed to thaw and repeated (two 'freeze/thaw' cycles). The patient should be told to expect blistering, followed by healing with crust formation. The lesion should separate within 3 weeks.

Benign tumours

Benign epidermal tumours

Seborrhoeic keratoses
Seborrhoeic keratoses (also known as seborrhoeic warts or basal cell papillomas) are very common. They are most frequently seen in elderly patients and may be solitary or multiple. Occasionally they run into hundreds, a tendency which may be familial. The head, neck, backs of the hands and forearms and the trunk are the sites of predilection.

Examination reveals a flat-topped area of skin with a 'stuck-on' appearance (Fig. 9.1). They are sometimes pale in colour, but are often pigmented and sometimes deeply so. The surface is often said to be rather greasy, but a more useful feature is the presence of small indentations and irregularities, which give the surface a granular look and feel.

The diagnosis is usually straightforward but very darkly pigmented lesions can be mistaken for malignant melanoma. On the face, seborrhoeic keratoses may remain virtually flat and there may be real difficulty in distinguishing them from senile lentigo or lentigo maligna (see below). Another diagnostic problem

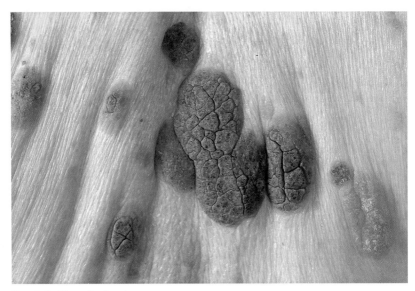

Fig. 9.1. Typical seborrhoeic warts.

can arise if lesions become inflamed through rubbing or other external trauma. There may be crusting and bleeding, and biopsy for histology may be necessary.

If treatment is deemed necessary (there is no malignant potential), the most satisfactory approach for smaller lesions is cryotherapy with liquid nitrogen, but larger ones may be better treated by curettage and cautery or even excision.

Skin tags (acrochordons)

Many people develop these small pedunculated lesions around the neck and axillae. Sometimes small melanocytic naevi may produce a similar appearance but most are more akin to seborrhoeic keratoses. They are commoner in the elderly and in the obese. They can be removed very easily with a cautery.

Keratoacanthoma

This tumour is an oddity. It used to be termed molluscum sebaceum. Some authors classify keratoacanthoma as malignant because histologically it looks like a squamous cell carcinoma (see below).

Clinically, the lesion arises rapidly, almost invariably on light-exposed skin. They are much commoner in the elderly. The lesion reaches a maximal size of a centimetre or two over the course of 6–8 weeks. A fully-formed tumour is seen in Fig. 9.2. As can be seen, it is round with rolled edges and a central keratin plug. The base is often red and inflamed, and the patient may complain that the lump is painful. Occasionally, a keratoacanthoma reaches a much greater size. The lesion eventually reaches a maximum and then begins to shrink in size, often almost as quickly as it enlarged. It finally disappears completely, leaving a small puckered scar.

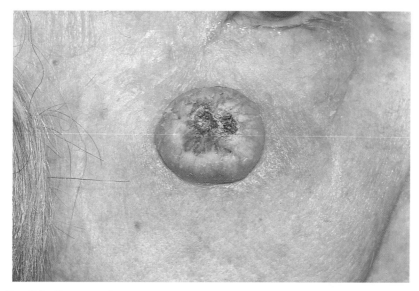

Fig. 9.2. Keratoacanthoma.

Although clinically somewhat similar, diagnostic differentiation from basal cell carcinoma (see below) can usually be made on the history of rapid growth and on the fact the lesion is so perfectly round. The main problem is to distinguish *prospectively* between a keratoacanthoma and a squamous cell carcinoma. By definition the keratoacanthoma is self-resolving, but this fact cannot be determined in advance. Incisional biopsies are generally unhelpful because of the close similarities between keratoacathoma and squamous cell carcinoma. It may be reasonable to wait expectantly for a few weeks if a lesion is considered to be very typical clinically, especially in the elderly or frail. However, if there is any diagnostic doubt these lesions are best removed by curettage or excision and sent for histology. Indeed it is probably simpler to remove a suspected keratoacanthoma while it is still small, rather than wait until a more complex procedure is required when it has become much larger.

Other benign epidermal tumours
Viral warts are dealt with in Chapter 3 and the other benign epidermal tumours listed are rare.

Epidermal cysts
There are three common forms of epidermal cyst. Two are usually called sebaceous cysts (a misnomer): the common scalp cyst, correctly termed a pilar or trichilemmal cyst, and the epidermoid cyst. Both are characterized histologically by the fact that the wall is composed of a modified epithelium.
    Pilar cysts are found on the scalp, are often multiple and may run in families. They may become huge and they often catch on combs or brushes.

Epidermoid cysts may be found anywhere but are most common on the head, neck and trunk. They often follow bad acne. The lesion consists of a cystic swelling within the skin and there may be an overlying punctum visible.

Both these types of cyst can be removed easily under local anaesthetic by a linear incision over the surface.

The third is the milium, an extremely common keratin cyst (Fig. 9.3). Milia may occur after trauma or blistering in the skin, or they may be spontaneous. In some families there is an inherited tendency to develop milia, especially in clusters on the cheeks and around the eyes. They can be treated by incision, pricking out or cautery.

Benign melanocytic tumours

Freckles and lentigines

These are both benign melanocytic lesions. We are all familiar with the freckles (ephelides) which are so common in red-heads. These are due to areas of skin containing melanocytes which are particularly responsive to stimulation by UV radiation. Lentigines are more permanent flat pigmented areas which are composed of increased numbers of melanocytes.

Melanocytic naevi are discussed in Chapter 10.

Benign dermal tumours

Dermatofibromas (or histiocytomas)

These are very common (Fig. 9.4). They are benign dermal lumps composed of fibrous tissue and some blood vessels. Usually found on the legs, and more

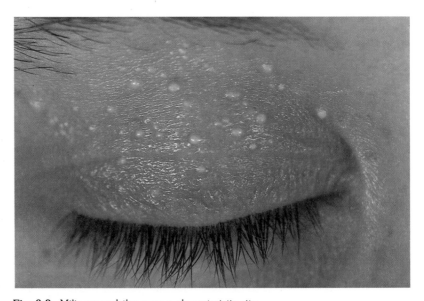

Fig. 9.3. Milia around the eyes: a characteristic site.

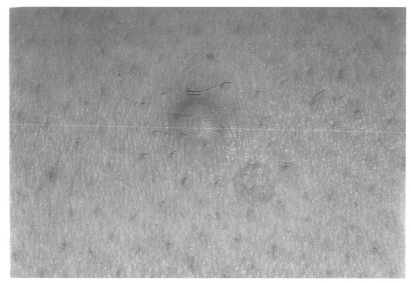

Fig. 9.4. Dermatofibroma (histiocytoma).

common in women, they may be easier to diagnose by touch than by sight: they feel like small lentils in the skin. Occasionally, they are heavily pigmented, which can cause diagnostic confusion. Excision may be cosmetically indicated.

Angioma

Angiomas of various kinds are seen. They are collections of aberrant blood vessels within the dermis and/or subcutaneous tissues. Some are developmental defects, commonly present at birth, and these are covered in Chapter 10. Others develop during adult life, such as the ubiquitous Campbell de Morgan spot (Fig. 9.5).

Pyogenic granuloma

Pyogenic granulomas are very common benign reactive inflammatory masses composed of blood vessels with a few fibroblasts. They erupt rapidly, often at the site of an injury or infection and usually have a polypoid appearance (Fig. 9.6), often with a 'collar' around the base. Profuse contact bleeding is a common presenting symptom. Their importance lies in the differential diagnosis from malignancies such as squamous carcinomas and melanomas. Removal by curettage or excision should therefore always be followed by histological confirmation.

Other dermal lumps that may be seen include neurofibromas, often in the context of Von Recklinghausen's neurofibromatosis, and other fibroblastic tumours. Fatty lumps (or lipomas) are lesions of subcutaneous tissue and are usually readily identified by their soft texture and lobulated outline. Occasionally, however, there may be difficulty distinguishing a lipoma from a diffuse dermal tumour or cyst.

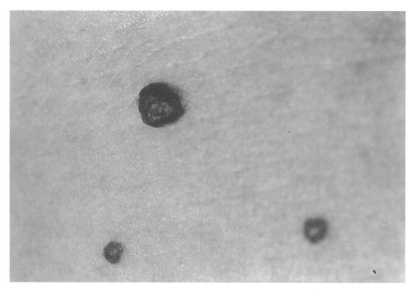

Fig. 9.5. Campbell de Morgan spots.

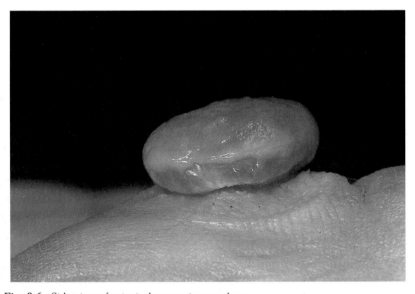

Fig. 9.6. Side view of a typical pyogenic granuloma.

Pseudotumours

Chondrodermatitis nodularis helicis

We mention this curious lesion here because it is often confused with basal cell carcinomas or other tumours. In reality, it is an inflammatory process and not a tumour at all. It presents as a small umbilicated nodule on the rim of the ear, usually in men (Fig. 9.7). The clue to the diagnosis is that it is painful, especially in bed at night. It can easily be excised.

Hypertrophic scars and keloids

Scar formation sometimes becomes very exuberant, resulting in protruberant masses of fibrous tissue. We consider the terms 'hypertrophic scar' and 'keloid', which are used to describe this, to be essentially the same, although some authors distinguish between them and would only use the latter term for lesions which spread laterally beyond the original wound (keloids can become very large). Keloids often itch.

Some sites are more prone to keloid formation: chest, upper back, shoulder, pubic region, ear lobes. They are much commoner in children and young adults and black skin is also more susceptible. Most follow known trauma, especially cuts (which may be surgical), ear-piercing, burns and acne. BCG inoculations performed high on the shoulder are another common cause. Some appear to develop spontaneously and can give rise to diagnostic confusion.

Excision generally leads to recurrence and management can be extremely difficult. Intralesional steroids, cryotherapy and radiotherapy before and after excision all have their advocates.

Dysplastic and malignant tumours

The term *dysplasia* in skin lesions implies a situation in which the skin has been partly or wholly replaced by cells which show neoplastic features when viewed under the microscope. When this results in invasion of adjacent tissue, the process can genuinely be said to be 'malignant'. Cutaneous dysplasias and malignancies are very common. Most are more frequent in ageing skin and in

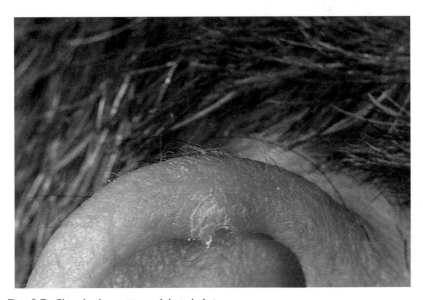

Fig. 9.7. Chondrodermatitis nodularis helicis.

skin which has been exposed to prolonged UV radiation. However, it is important to note that there are other factors which are associated with dysplastic skin changes. Most forms of ionizing radiation other than UV (e.g. X-rays, γ-rays) are also powerful inducers of skin cancer. There are a number of known topical carcinogens. Exposure to some industrial oils, tars and bitumen has been associated with skin cancers, as was chronic exposure to soot in chimney sweeps, which resulted in scrotal cancers. Skin cancers are also a feature of a number of genetic diseases. A notable example is xeroderma pigmentosum, in which repair mechanisms of UV-induced DNA damage are faulty. This leads to multiple tumours of various cell types.

In this section we shall review the features of the most common and important cutaneous dysplastic and malignant skin tumours.

Dysplastic/malignant epidermal tumours

Actinic or solar keratoses

These are common and consist of areas of dysplastic epithelium. They tend to be red and scaly patches (Fig. 9.8) in which, characteristically, the intensity of both features varies with time. They are seen on light-exposed skin, especially the face, forearms, dorsa of hands, the lower legs and on the bald scalp. In heavily sun-exposed individuals there may be many hundreds of lesions, and they also become more numerous with increasing age. Some actinic keratoses become pigmented, which can lead to diagnostic confusion with lentigo maligna (see below).

Actinic keratoses have malignant potential, albeit relatively small. They should in general be treated, although in the very elderly or when there are

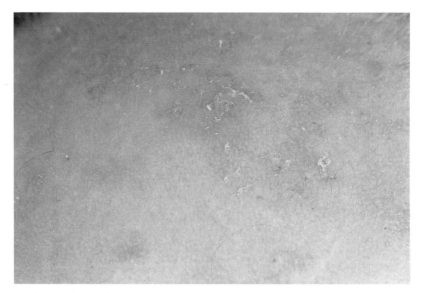

Fig. 9.8. Multiple solar keratoses.

many lesions this may be impractical. The treatment of choice is cryotherapy, but large areas on the face and scalp can be treated with the topical antimitotic agent 5-fluorouracil.

Squamous cell carcinoma in situ or Bowen's disease

Bowen's disease represents squamous cell carcinoma in which the dysplastic changes remain confined to the epidermis. There is no invasive component. The condition usually presents as a solitary patch of red scaly skin, although multiple patches may also occur. There is a superficial resemblance to psoriasis (Fig. 9.9), but the surface scale is adherent rather than flaky, as it is in psoriasis. Furthermore, removal of the scale leaves a glistening red surface which does not usually bleed. Like the other epidermal dysplasias, lesions are more common in the elderly and on light-exposed skin. It is important to note, however, that Bowen's disease may occur on non-exposed areas such as the trunk. Previous arsenic therapy may predispose to multiple areas of Bowen's disease and superficial basal cell carcinomas (see below). Since arsenic was in a number of tonics and was used in the past for psoriasis, it is important to keep an eye open for possible Bowen's disease in the elderly, especially if psoriatic.

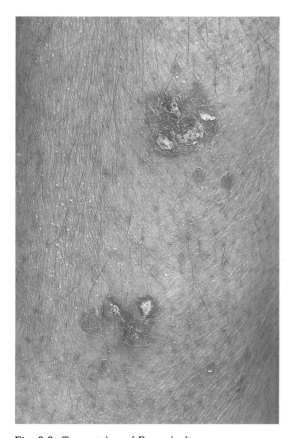

Fig. 9.9. Two patches of Bowen's disease.

Bowen's disease is not normally symptomatic and is not steroid-responsive. Although change to invasive carcinoma is rare, Bowen's disease should be treated by curettage or cryotherapy. Very large areas may require radiotherapy.

The same dysplastic changes may occur on the penis, where the clinical appearance is usually of a velvety red plaque. This change is termed erythroplasia of Queyrat, but it has the same significance as Bowen's disease elsewhere.

Another condition which produces a clinically similar change is Paget's disease (Fig. 9.10). This should always be suspected if a unilateral scaly red patch on the nipple fails to respond to topical steroids and a biopsy may be necessary. There is always an underlying carcinoma for which mastectomy is required.

Invasive squamous cell carcinoma

Squamous cell carcinoma is a serious matter. Lesions may metastasize to local lymph nodes and beyond, particularly those in and around the mouth or genitalia.

Squamous cell carcinomas of the skin present in a number of clinical guises: (i) they may be keratotic lumps, which can be very difficult to distinguish from a hypertrophic actinic keratosis without a biopsy; (ii) they may appear as rapidly growing polypoid masses (Fig. 9.11); and (iii) as cutaneous ulcers. These tumours arise commonly on aged and sun-damaged skin and are often surrounded by actinic keratoses. Squamous cell carcinomas also develop on the lips and in the mouth (Fig. 9.12), where smoking is an important aetiological factor. Lesions may also appear on the genitalia, in which initiation by human papilloma virus is increasingly important.

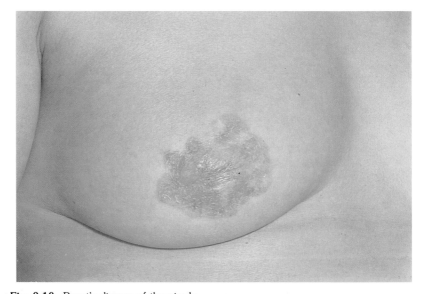

Fig. 9.10. Paget's disease of the nipple.

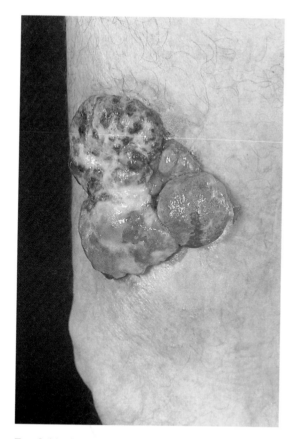

Fig. 9.11. A polypoid squamous cell carcinoma.

Squamous cell carcinomas are best removed where possible. Alternatively, radiotherapy may be used following a biopsy to confirm the diagnosis.

Basal cell carcinomas

These are by far the commonest malignant skin tumours and are often known to the general public as 'rodent ulcers'. Most are seen on the face, but they do occur on other sun-exposed sites. They may also appear in the hair-bearing scalp, behind the ear and on the trunk. The majority of basal cell carcinomas begin as a nodule which spreads slowly outwards, usually leaving a central depression (Fig. 9.13). It is this progression which creates the classical 'rolled edge'. The tumour is usually skin-coloured and has a slightly translucent look—often described as 'pearly'. A very characteristic feature is the presence of telangietatic vessels on the surface (Fig. 9.13). This accounts for a frequent presenting complaint in basal cell carcinomas of contact bleeding.

There are also several distinctive clinical variants of the basal cell carcinoma which should be mentioned. Some tumours adopt a flat growth pattern which results in a scar-like appearance. This is known as the *morphoeic* or *cicatrizing* basal cell carcinoma. This type of tumour can cause particular diagnostic

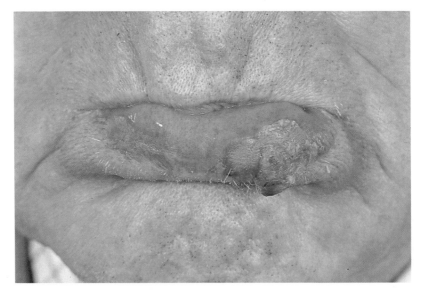

Fig. 9.12. Squamous cell carcinoma on the lip.

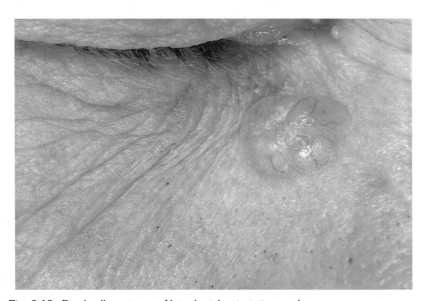

Fig. 9.13. Basal cell carcinoma. Note the telangiectatic vessels.

problems and it is also difficult to assess where the tumour begins and ends. On the trunk, a *superficial* growth pattern is very common (Fig. 9.14). These lesions may grow for many years and can reach a size many centimetres across. They are usually solitary, but multiple superficial basal cell carcinomas, like Bowen's disease (see above), may be associated with previous arsenic ingestion. The diagnosis can be difficult, and lesions are often treated as inflammatory. However, on careful inspection, a fine, 'wormy' edge is generally visible, which

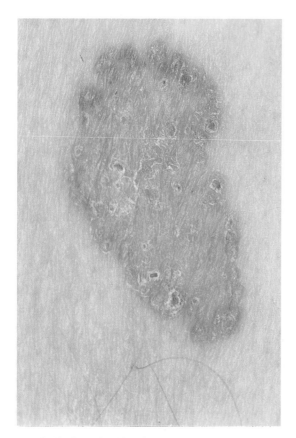

Fig. 9.14. Superficial basal carcinoma.

is often flecked with pigment. Basal cell carcinomas generally may be *pigmented*. This is usually patchy and relatively mild, but heavily pigmented lesions do occur and these may cause diagnostic confusion.

The treatment of basal cell carcinomas may be by excision, biopsy and radiotherapy or, in the case of superficial tumours, curettage or cryotherapy. Fortunately, mestastases from basal cell carcinomas are extremely rare. However, the tumour is locally invasive and can be very destructive (Fig. 9.15). This is especially true of the morphoeic variant. It is also particularly important to deal adequately with lesions around the eyes, nose and ears, because the tumour can spread along the bony passages into the skull.

Dysplastic/malignant melanocytic tumours

Lentigo maligna

Lentigo maligna (or Hutchinson's malignant freckle) is the name given to a patch of proliferating, malignant melanocytes which occurs on sun-damaged skin. This proliferation is radial and often lasts for many years, but an invasive nodular component may develop at any time. Clinically, there is a flat, brown

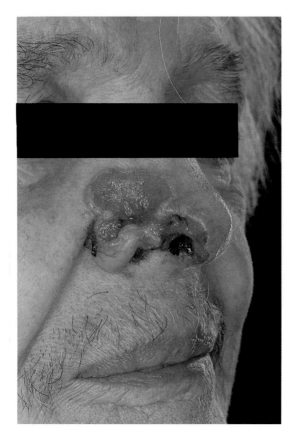

Fig. 9.15. Basal cell carcinoma. Such destruction gives rise to the term 'rodent ulcer'.

area with irregular pigmentation, usually on the cheek or forehead (Fig. 9.16). These can be difficult to distinguish clinically from flat seborrhoeic warts, pigmented actinic keratoses and simple lentigos. A biopsy is essential if there is any doubt. Treatment is a matter of some debate. Most dermatologists now freeze the area with liquid nitrogen, but if the lesion is small it can be excised. In the very elderly, it may also be reasonable to leave it alone and simply follow the patient up carefully.

Malignant melanoma

This is the most dangerous of the malignant skin tumours. There are four recognized patterns of malignant melanoma:

1 *Lentigo maligna melanoma* This is the name given to the appearance of a nodule of invasive melanoma within a lentigo maligna (see above).

2 *Superficial spreading melanoma* This is the commonest in the UK. Although most frequently on the legs in women and the trunk in men, these lesions may appear anywhere. They are irregularly pigmented brown/black patches with an irregular edge (Fig. 9.17). They often itch or give rise to mild discomfort.

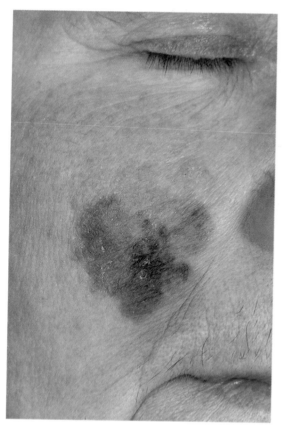

Fig. 9.16. Lentigo maligna.

3 *Nodular melanomas* These present as rapidly growing lumps anywhere on the body surface (Fig. 9.18) Occasionally they are warty (verrucous melanoma) or non-pigmented (amelanotic melanoma) and these types are especially difficult to diagnose.

4 *Acral melanoma* This is rare in the UK. It is, however, much more common in other countries (e.g. Japan) and is, for example, virtually the only type of melanoma seen in UK residents of Asian or Afro-Caribbean origin. Acral melanoma may present as a pigmented patch on the hand or foot, where the main differential diagnosis is from a viral wart. Alternatively, this tumour may appear as an area of subungual pigmentation. The decision as to whether such a lesion is a haematoma or a melanocytic lesion can be very difficult.

Melanomas, other than lentigo maligna melanoma, occur in a relatively younger age group than basal or squamous cell carcinomas. The incidence of melanoma is rising rapidly, even in temperate climates. It is thought that this is at least partly related to the increase in intermittent sun exposure that has occurred since it became cosmetically fashionable to be tanned. Rising

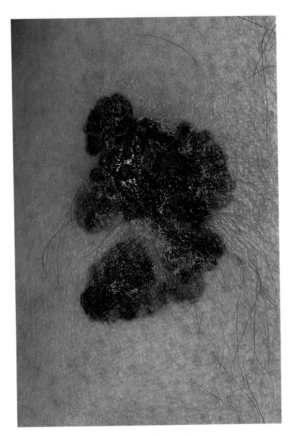

Fig. 9.17. Superficial spreading melanoma.

standards of living have permitted more and more people from northern climes to take brief sunny holidays abroad (and at home), during which one of the most important 'activities' has been sunbathing. It seems that such intermittent periods of exposure to strong sunlight (and possibly episodes of sunburn) are particularly risky. There is also disturbing evidence that such sun exposure in childhood may be particularly important. All of us have seen children in gardens, around pools and on the beach being allowed to run about with little or nothing on. Where this used mostly to be in the home country it is now increasingly possible for families to spend 2 or 3 weeks each year in areas such as the Mediterranean, Florida or even further afield. It is important to note, too, that 25–50% of melanomas arise in pre-existing melanocytic naevi (see Chapter 10). It seems that the incidence of this varies from country to country.

The prognosis of malignant melanoma can be related accurately to the depth to which the tumour cells have invaded at the time of first excision. It does not matter whether the tumour was initially superficial spreading, nodular or either of the other types described above. Most centres now measure the

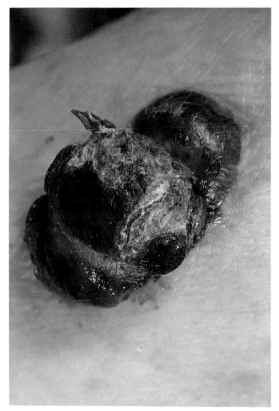

Fig. 9.18. Large nodular melanoma.

depth of invasion using a technique known as the Breslow thickness (Fig. 9.19). If the tumour is < 1.5 mm at first excision the 5-year survival rate is in the order of 90%. If the tumour has invaded to a depth > 3.5 mm, however, the 5-year survival figure is about 40%.

The treatment of all types of melanoma, other than lentigo maligna and diagnostically difficult acral lesions where an incisional biopsy may be justified, is excision as soon as possible. There is a debate about how wide such an excision should be and the practice will vary from area to area and from surgeon to surgeon. There is no harm, however, in an initial narrow excision margin. The urgency is to remove the melanoma and to worry about further procedures later.

Surgery is the only satisfactory treatment. Radiotherapy and chemotherapy have little to offer at present. Because the prognosis of malignant melanoma relates directly to depth of invasion of the tumour, it is also important that patients with melanoma present for treatment as soon as possible. In many countries attempts have been made to try and encourage the public to keep an eye open for possible malignant melanomas.

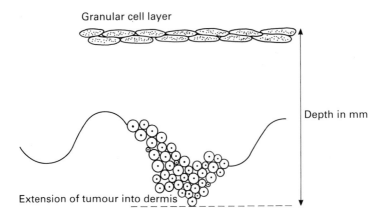

Fig. 9.19. Breslow thickness.

Many doctors also use a checklist for suspicious pigmented lesions similar to the following:

1 Is an existing mole getting larger or a new one growing? After puberty moles usually do not grow. (This sign essentially refers to adults. Remember that naevi may grow rapidly in children—see Chapter 10.)

2 Does the lesion have an irregular outline? Ordinary moles are a smooth, regular shape.

3 Is the lesion irregularly pigmented? Particularly, is there a mixture of shades of brown and black?

4 Is the lesion > 1 cm in diameter?

5 Is the lesion inflamed or is there a reddish edge?

6 Is the lesion bleeding, oozing or crusting?

7 Does the lesion itch or hurt?

Any pigmented lesion, whether newly arising or already present, which exhibits three or more of these features, especially the first three, should be treated as highly suspicious.

Prevention of epithelial and melanocytic malignancies

Genetic and constitutional factors are important in determining whether an individual develops skin cancer. Both types of epithelial skin cancers and melanomas are more common in those who burn easily in the sun: those with fair skin, fair or red hair and blue or green eyes (Skin Types I and II—see Chapter 15). Melanomas are also more common in individuals with many melanocytic naevi.

However, it is also quite apparent that chronic exposure to UV radiation is associated with basal and squamous cell carcinomas and there is a great deal of evidence which also links melanoma to UV radiation. It seems logical, therefore, to recommend that those at greatest risk should avoid excessive sun exposure. No fair-skinned individual should allow him or herself to get sunburnt. It is probably best for them to keep out of the sun during the middle of the day (between 11.00 h and 15.00 h) as far as possible. They should also wear sun screens with a high degree of barrier function. Those who tan easily and those with genetically brown or black skin need not take such Draconian precautions but sun exposure in all children should be similarly restricted. Whether such advice will be widely taken up remains to be seen.

Dysplasic/dermal malignant tumours

Malignant sarcomas may develop in the skin. They usually present as indolent nodules which grow relatively slowly, but become fixed to deeper tissues. The diagnosis is made by biopsy and further wide excision is generally required. In one low-grade tumour of this kind—dermatofibrosarcoma protruberans—such excision needs to be very wide indeed.

Kaposi's sarcoma

This malignant vascular tumour merits special mention in spite of its rarity. Kaposi's sarcoma was first described among Ashkenazi Jews in whom the disease pursues a low-grade course. Pigmented patches and purplish plaques appear on the legs and slowly progress. A similar pattern is seen amongst

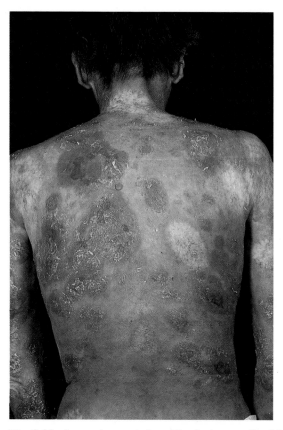

Fig. 9.20. Areas of mycosis fungoides (cutaneous T cell lymphoma).

northern Italians. However, a much more aggressive form of the disease has been observed in Africa and multiple nodules of Kaposi's sarcoma occur in patients with the acquired immunodeficiency syndrome (AIDS).

Lymphomas

Occasionally the skin is the site of lymphomatous malignancy. This may be secondary to lymphoma elsewhere, as is usually the case if a non-Hodgkin's B cell lymphoma infiltrates the skin. However, the skin may be the original site of lymphomatous change, especially in cutaneous T cell lymphoma (often called 'mycosis fungoides'). In this condition, an aberrant clone of T lymphocytes appears to develop. A variety of skin changes result, many of which remain unchanged or grow only very slowly for many years. Ultimately, however, the process becomes more actively proliferative, and plaques and tumours may develop. These lesions are red, well-circumscribed and scaly and can be confused with psoriasis (Fig. 9.20). The definitive diagnosis is reached by biopsy. Eventually, T cell invasion of lymph nodes and other organs occurs. Treatment is difficult and may involve UV radiation with or without psoralens, radiotherapy, and chemotherapy with cytotoxics. The choice depends on the stage of the disease.

Extension from deeper tissues and metastases

It should not be forgotten that tumours of underlying structures, such as breast, may invade the skin. The skin may also be the site of metastatic deposits from internal cancers such as bronchogenic carcinoma (see Chapter 19).

Chapter 10
Naevi

Ten thousand saw I at a glance
(William Wordsworth;
I wandered lonely as a Cloud)

Naevi are extremely common—virtually everyone has some. But what is a naevus? The most appropriate definition is that the word 'naevus' represents a cutaneous hamartoma, i.e. a lesion in which essentially normal tissue components are present in abnormal quantities or patterns. This allows for those naevi which are not actually present at birth, and develop during childhood or even later, but which arise from cells which were present during intrauterine life.

However, this term has given rise to much confusion over the years. In classical times it seems to have been used rather loosely, meaning almost any lump or wart, and unfortunately the same often applies today. Much of the difficulty arises from the fact that the term has been used in several different ways, in addition to that defined above. For example, some writers use the word without qualification to mean the commonest of cutaneous hamartomas, the melanocytic naevus (see below). The word is also applied to lesions which are unrelated to congenital defects, such as the so-called 'spider naevus' (which should properly be called a 'spider telangiectasis').

The situation is complicated by the fact that some lesions which are certainly 'naevi' are also given a variety of other names such as 'mole' or 'birthmark', especially by patients, but that these words are used inaccurately. For example, a lump described as a 'mole' may be a melanocytic naevus, but it may also be any small skin lesion, especially if it is pigmented. The term 'birthmark' is accurate enough as far as it goes, but many true naevi are not present at birth.

In this chapter, we shall use the term 'naevus' as outlined in the first definition. We shall also use the term 'naevoid' to describe apparently congenital naevus-like malformations. The constituents of a naevus may arise from any component of the skin and naevi may be classified accordingly (Table 10.1). In this chapter, however, we need to discuss in detail only the most important: epithelial and organoid naevi, vascular naevi and melanocytic naevi.

Epithelial and 'organoid' naevi

These are developmental defects which derive from epidermal structures, such as epidermis itself, hair follicles and sebaceous glands. They are generally rare, but there are two important types that should be mentioned briefly:

Table 10.1. Constituents of a naevus

Epithelial/'organoid'
  Epidermal
  Sebaceous
  Hair follicle

Melanocytic
  Congenital
    Congenital melanocytic naevus
    Mongolian blue spot
  Acquired
    Junctional/compound/intradermal
    Sutton's halo naevus
    Dysplastic naevus
    Spitz naevus
    Blue naevus

Vascular
  Telangiectatic
    Superficial capillary
    Deep capillary
    Rare telangiectatic disorders
  Angiomatous

Other tissues
  Connective tissue
  Mast cell
  Fat

Epidermal naevus

These are circumscribed areas of epidermal thickening. They are present at birth or develop during early childhood. They are often linear (Fig. 10.1). Very rarely, there are associated CNS abnormalities.

Another type of epidermal naevus is the so-called *Becker's naevus*. This is a pigmented hairy patch which develops at or around puberty on the upper trunk or shoulder of young men.

Sebaceous naevus

Sebaceous naevi are usually present at birth, but may be overlooked. They present as flat, slightly yellow areas. They are nearly always on the head and neck and, if they are in the scalp, can give rise to a localized area of alopecia. As time passes, the naevus becomes thickened and warty. The importance of these lesions is that basal cell carcinomas may arise within them in later life. They are best excised during adolescence.

Melanocytic naevi

These are by far the commonest of the naevi. They are formed from melanocytes which have failed to mature or migrate properly during embryonic development. Almost all of us have some and many of us have many of this type of naevus. We need therefore only look at our own skin to see typical examples.

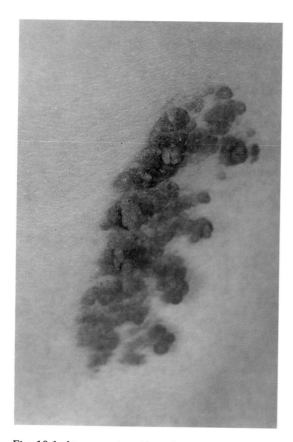

Fig. 10.1. Linear warty epidermal naevus.

It is convenient to subdivide melanocytic naevi into certain specific categories (*see above*), based on clinical and histopathological features because there are some relevant differences between them. The first important difference is whether or not they are present at birth (congenital) or arise later (acquired).

Congenital

Congenital melanocytic naevus

About 1% of children are born with a melanocytic naevus already present. These may vary in size from only a few millimetres to many centimetres. Occasionally a child is born with a huge, grossly disfiguring variant, known as the giant congenital melanocytic or 'bathing trunk' naevus (Fig. 10.2). It has been said that congenital melanocytic naevi are more prone to develop melanomas than acquired lesions, and this is certainly true of the giant type. Furthermore, the very rare prepubertal malignant melanomas that are encountered are nearly always seen in a congenital naevus. However, it is not known how often malignancy develops in smaller congenital melanocytic naevi.

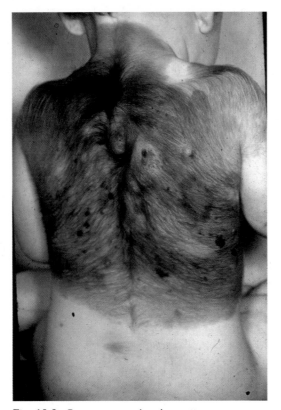

Fig. 10.2. Giant congenital melanocytic naevus.

There is a paradox in the management of these tumours. Small, low-risk naevi can be removed easily but larger lesions, which may have a higher malignant potential, may require extensive, even mutilating, surgery. Each case must therefore be judged on its own merits, with decisions being taken by all concerned including the child and its parents.

Mongolian blue spot

Mongolian blue spot is the name given to naevoid lesions found in many children of Mongoloid or Indian extraction, usually in a diffuse patch on the lower back and buttocks (Fig. 10.3). As in blue naevi (see below), the colour is due to the presence of melanocytes in the dermis, but these are more widely dispersed. The areas are present at birth but generally fade as the child grows up, but they may persist indefinitely. Unwary casualty officers have occasionally mistaken Mongolian blue spots for bruising and accused parents of baby-battering.

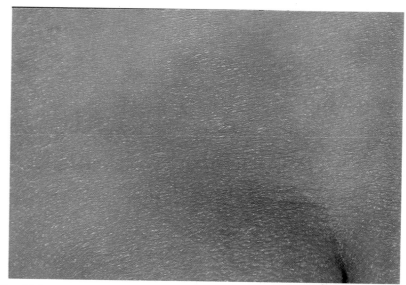

Fig. 10.3. Mongolian blue spot.

Acquired

Acquired melanocytic naevus

A melanocytic naevus is said to be 'acquired' if it is not present at birth but develops during post-natal life. This type of naevus is extremely common and is generally accepted as a 'normal' feature. Indeed at some points in history so-called 'beauty spots' were highly fashionable. At worst, most only represent a minor cosmetic nuisance.

The first thing to make clear in considering naevi of this kind is that each naevus has its own sequential life history. This will make it easier to understand the terms which are applied to the different stages in their evolutionary process. These are illustrated graphically in Fig. 10.4.

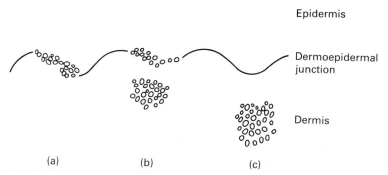

Fig. 10.4. The phases of the acquired melanocytic naevus: (a) junctional; (b) compound; and (c) intradermal.

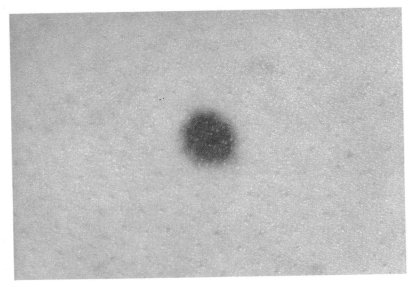

Fig. 10.5. Acquired melanocytic naevus.

An acquired melanocytic naevus (Fig. 10.5) first becomes noticeable when a group of immature melanocytes begins to proliferate at the dermoepidermal junction. After a period of horizontal growth along the dermoepidermal junction, some of the cells migrate down into the dermis. Eventually all the melanocytic cells are confined to the dermis. Lesions at each of these phases are called, respectively: *junctional* naevi, *compound* naevi and *intradermal* naevi. Different melanocytic naevi will be at different stages of development in the same individual.

The majority of melanocytic naevi begin to appear in the first 20 years of life, but some may continue to develop into the 30s and 40s. Early in life they are pigmented, often heavily so, but later they may become quite pale, especially when completely intradermal. Eventually, most disappear altogether. Very few octogenarians have many melanocytic naevi.

The importance of these naevi lies in the fact that up to 50% of malignant melanomas develop within a pre-existing naevus, although the chances of this happening to any one lesion are infinitesimally small. However, it is known that the possession of a large number of acquired melanocytic naevi is a significant risk factor for melanoma. No-one is entirely sure what triggers malignant change in a naevus but much of the epidemiological evidence points to a link with UV exposure.

It is obviously important that any melanocytic naevus that begins to behave oddly is removed immediately and examined histologically, but it is also important to remember that, by definition, all melanocytic naevi grow at some stage. Growth alone, therefore, is not necessarily a sinister sign, especially in younger individuals. Most naevi undergoing malignant change will exhibit several of the features outlined in the list on p. 128, such as alteration in pigmentation, irregularity of the edge, inflammation, itch or bleeding. However, if there is any doubt excision is the best policy.

In addition to the 'ordinary' type of melanocytic naevus described above, there are several variants that deserve a special mention:

Sutton's halo naevus

Occasionally an otherwise typical acquired melanocytic naevus develops a white ring around it, becomes red and undergoes spontaneous regression (Fig. 10.6). This bizarre reaction is an immune response to the naevus, the reason for which is unknown. It is of no sinister significance. The white patch usually repigments rapidly.

Dysplastic naevus

The term 'dysplasia' in relation to skin lesions is discussed in Chapter 2. The concept of the 'dysplastic' melanocytic naevus is a relatively new one. Although some authorities believe that such lesions can be distinguished clinically, the basic criteria for the diagnosis of a 'dysplastic' naevus are histopathological and are beyond the scope of this book. However, it is not all that uncommon for an

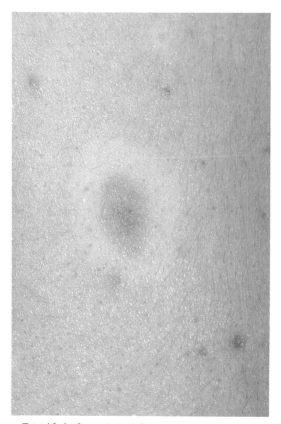

Fig. 10.6. Sutton's 'halo' naevus.

active-looking junctional melanocytic naevus to be removed and for the pathology report to record some 'dysplastic' features.

The importance of this type of naevus is that some families have an autosomal dominant disorder characterized by multiple dysplastic naevi and a high incidence of malignant melanoma.

Blue naevus

These lesions have a predilection for the extremities, head and buttocks. Their characteristic slate-blue colour (Fig. 10.7) is due to the deep position of pigment-producing melanocytes in the dermis.

Spitz naevus

This lesion is also known as *juvenile melanoma*, with or without the prefix 'benign'. This term is, however, best dropped because it simply causes confusion. It is a benign lesion of children which has a characteristic brick-red colour, due to a prominent vascular component in the naevus. The importance of Spitz naevi lies in the fact that histologically they can be confused with a malignant melanoma.

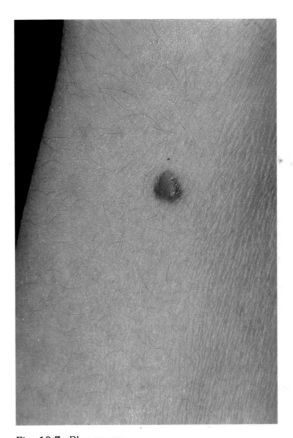

Fig. 10.7. Blue naevus.

Vascular naevi

Vascular naevi are common. Some present relatively minor problems, while others can be very disfiguring. The subclassification of this type of naevus is confusing and by no means uniform. We have adopted a relatively simple approach based on both clinical and pathological features.

Telangiectatic naevi

Superficial capillary naevus

These are extremely common pink, flat areas composed of dilated capillaries in the superficial dermis (Fig. 10.8). They are found in about 50% of all neonates. The commonest site is the nape of the neck, where they may be called 'salmon patches' or 'stork marks'. Other affected sites include the forehead and glabellar region ('stork marks' again) and the eyelids ('angel's kisses'). Most facial lesions fade, but those on the neck often persist into adult life, although they are usually hidden by hair.

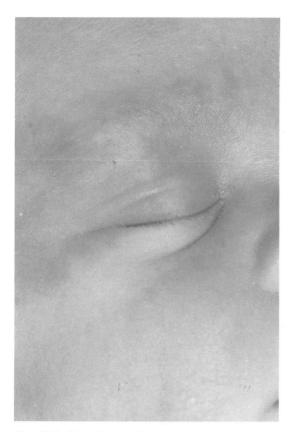

Fig. 10.8. Superficial capillary naevus.

Deep capillary naevus

These lesions are often called 'port-wine stains' or 'port-wine marks'. Dilated capillaries are present in the upper dermis, but also appear at deeper levels. The deeper component gradually extends during life.

Deep capillary naevi are much rarer but are more important cosmetically than the superficial types described above. They also present at birth, and may vary in colour from a pale pink to deep purple. The lesions are most often seen on the head and neck and are usually unilateral, often appearing to follow the territory of one or more branches of the trigeminal nerve (Fig. 10.9). They may be only a few centimetres across or they may be very extensive. If a deep capillary naevus is relatively pale in colour it may be difficult to distinguish from the superficial type, especially in the neonatal period. It is therefore important to give a somewhat guarded initial prognosis and await events.

Unlike superficial capillary naevi, deep lesions show no tendency to fade. Indeed the intensity of the colour deepens with time and the affected area may also become progressively thickened. Lumpy, angiomatous nodules may develop. This may be most unattractive and patients often seek help in improving the appearance. Sadly this is not always very successful, although

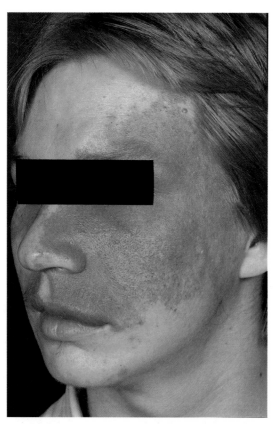

Fig. 10.9. Deep capillary naevus ('port-wine stain').

laser therapy can sometimes produce reasonable results. There is now a wide range of skin-coloured cosmetics which can be used to camouflage the lesions.

There are two important complications of 'port-wine'-type naevi:

1 There may be an associated intracranial vascular malformation which may result in fits, long tract signs and mental retardation. This is known as the *Sturge–Weber syndrome.*

2 Congenital glaucoma may develop without other signs of the Sturge–Weber syndrome, especially in lesions involving the area of the ophthalmic nerve. Growth of underlying tissues may be abnormal with very deep lesions, resulting in hypertrophy of whole limbs—haemangiectatic hypertrophy.

Rare telangiectatic naevoid conditions

There are some rare conditions in which telangiectatic naevi appear and which deserve a brief mention. Little girls are occasionally seen with an area stippled with pin-point red or purple puncta. These blanch on pressure. This is known as *angioma serpiginosum.*

Multiple telangiectases on the face, mouth and hands may accompany internal lesions in *hereditary haemorrhagic telangiectasia* (see Chapter 11). Telangiectases are also a characteristic feature of another congenital disease *ataxia telangiectasia*, in which repeated infections and cerebellar ataxia also occur.

Telangiectatic areas with superficial hyperkeratosis may also be encountered. These are known as *angiokeratomas.* Widespread lesions of this type develop in the inherited disorder *Anderson–Fabry disease.*

Angiomatous naevi

These naevi are thicker from the outset than the capillary type. Most authorities acknowledge that they usually contain both capillary-derived elements as well as larger, so-called 'cavernous' vascular spaces. In some accounts, these lesions are classified as capillary, while in others they are called cavernous angiomas.

Strawberry naevus

By far the most important of the angiomatous naevi is the so-called strawberry naevus. These arise very shortly after birth. They may appear anywhere but have a predilection for the head and neck and the napkin area (Fig. 10.10). They are usually solitary but occasionally there may be more than one. The lesion grows rapidly to produce a dome-shaped, red/purple extrusion which may bleed if traumatized. The vast majority reach a maximum size within a few months. They can be very large and unsightly.

Fortunately, most also undergo spontaneous resolution. Sometimes this begins with central necrosis of the lump, which can look very alarming (Fig. 10.10). It is said that 50% are gone by age 5 and 70% by age 7. Some, however, only regress partially and a few not at all. There is then a need for plastic surgical intervention.

The management of these lesions, in all but a few instances, is expectant. It is useful to be able to show the parents of a child with a strawberry naevus a

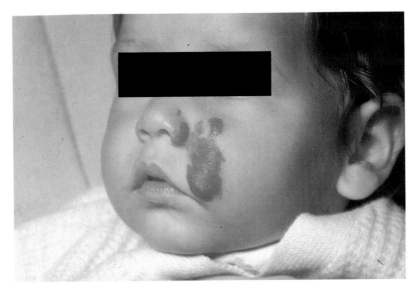

Fig. 10.10. Cavernous haemangiomas: Face.

series of pictures of previous patients in whom the lesion has gone. There are, however, some specific indications for intervention:

1 If the tumour obstructs breathing or feeding.

2 If the tumour occludes an *eye*, as this will lead to blindness in the affected eye.

3 If *severe* bleeding occurs.

4 If platelet sequestration occurs within the tumour leading to consumption coagulopathy *(Kasabach–Merritt syndrome)*.

5 If the tumour is still large and unsightly after the age of 10.

Most dermatologists would initially treat patients with the first four listed complications with high-dose prednisolone. This may produce a marked shrinkage of the naevus. If this fails, and in the fifth complication, complex surgical intervention may be required.

Rare angiomatous naevi

Rarely, infants are born with multiple angiomas of skin and internal organs. The skin lesions look like small strawberry naevi. This is known as *neonatal angiomatosis*. The prognosis is often poor.

Another rare naevus is the verrucous haemangioma, in which lesions of the deep angiomatous type develop secondary hyperkeratosis over the surface.

Other naevi

Naevi may be composed of other skin elements, including connective tissue, mast cells and fat. Although these are all rare, they may occasionally be seen. For example, the cutaneous stigmas of tuberous sclerosis are connective tissue naevi (See chapter 11).

Chapter 11
Inherited Disorders

> There is only one more beautiful thing than a fine healthy skin, and that is a rare skin disease.
>
> (Sir Erasmus Wilson, 1809–84)

Included in this chapter are a number of conditions which are known to be inherited in an autosomal dominant, autosomal recessive, X-linked recessive, or X-linked dominant pattern. Many of these disorders are rare, and are therefore only briefly mentioned. There are a number of skin diseases in which genetic factors play an important part, such as atopic eczema, psoriasis, acne vulgaris and male pattern balding, which are not discussed here, but described elsewhere in the book.

The ichthyoses

The term ichthyosis is derived from the Greek *ikhthus*, meaning fish, as the appearance of the skin has been likened to fish scales. The ichthyoses are a group of disorders of keratinization in which the skin is extremely dry and scaly (Fig. 11.1). In the majority of cases the disease is inherited, but occasionally ichthyosis may develop as an acquired phenomenon, for example in association with a lymphoma. There are several types of ichthyosis, with different patterns of inheritance.

Autosomal dominant ichthyosis (ichthyosis vulgaris)

This is the commonest type of ichthyosis, and is often quite mild. The skin is normal at birth, and scaling usually appears during early childhood. The skin on the trunk and extensor aspects of the limbs is dry and flaky, but the limb flexures are often spared. Dominant ichthyosis is frequently associated with an atopic constitution.

X-linked ichthyosis

This type of ichthyosis only affects males. The scales are larger and darker in colour than those of dominant ichthyosis, and usually the trunk and limbs are extensively involved, including the flexures. Corneal opacities may be seen on slit-lamp examination of affected individuals and carrier females, but these do not interfere with vision. Affected individuals are deficient in the enzyme steroid sulphatase, and this is thought to be related to the pathogenesis of the ichthyosis, although the precise mechanism is not known.

Both X-linked ichthyosis and autosomal dominant ichthyosis improve during the summer months.

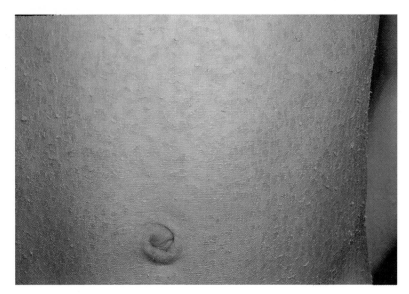

Fig. 11.1. Ichthyosis.

Ichthyosiform erythroderma
A bullous form of this condition is dominantly inherited, and a non-bullous form recessively inherited. In both conditions the skin is scaly and erythematous and often has an offensive odour.

Treatment
Treatment consists of the regular use of emollients and bath oils. Urea-containing creams are also helpful. The more severe types of ichthyosis often respond to oral therapy with the aromatic retinoid etretinate (Tigason).

Collodion baby
This terminology is applied to babies born encased in a transparent rigid membrane (Fig. 11.2). The membrane cracks and peels off after a few days. Some affected babies have an underlying ichthyotic disorder such as X-linked ichthyosis or ichthyosiform erythroderma, but many subsequently have a perfectly normal skin. Collodion babies have increased transepidermal water loss. They should be nursed in a high humidity environment and given additional oral fluids.

Palmoplantar keratoderma
There are several rare disorders in which there is massive thickening of the horny layer of the palms and soles. The commonest type of palmoplantar keratoderma is dominantly inherited. Many medical texts mention the association of palmoplantar keratoderma (tylosis) with carcinoma of the oesophagus—in fact this association has been recorded in only two families.

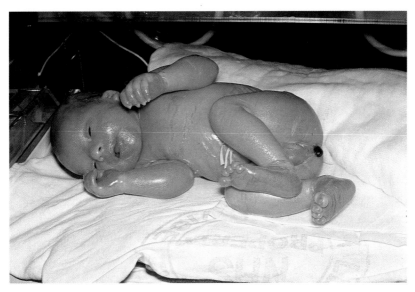

Fig. 11.2. Collodion baby.

Darier's disease (keratosis follicularis)

This is a dominantly inherited abnormality of keratinization which is usually first evident in late childhood or adolescence. The characteristic lesions of Darier's disease are brown follicular keratotic papules which are grouped together over the face and neck, the centre of the chest and back, the axillae and the groins (Fig. 11.3). The nails in Darier's disease typically show longitudinal pink or white bands, with V-shaped notches at the free edges of the nail plates. There are usually multiple plane wart-like lesions on the dorsa of the hands (acrokeratosis verruciformis).

Treatment

Darier's disease responds well to treatment with the retinoid etretinate (Tigason).

Epidermolysis bullosa

This group of hereditary blistering diseases is described in Chapter 14.

Ehlers–Danlos syndrome

There are a number of distinct variants of this condition, all of which are associated with abnormalities of collagen, principally defective production of certain collagen types. The most common variants are inherited in an autosomal dominant manner, but all types of Ehlers–Danlos syndrome are rare. Typical features are skin hyperextensibility and fragility and joint hypermobility. In certain types there is a risk of rupture of major blood vessels because of deficient collagen content in the vessel wall.

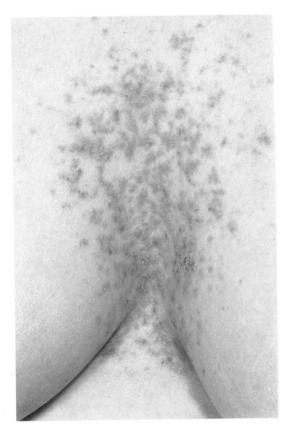

Fig. 11.3. Darier's disease.

Tuberous sclerosis (Epiloia)

This disorder is dominantly inherited, but many cases are the result of new mutations. Tuberous sclerosis is a condition in which there are hamartomatous malformations in the skin and internal organs. The characteristic skin lesions include numerous pink papules on the face (Fig. 11.4)—these were originally mistakenly called adenoma sebaceum, but are in fact hamartomas of connective tissue and small blood vessels (angiofibromas); the shagreen patch on the back (a connective tissue naevus); periungal fibromas (Fig. 11.5) and hypopigmented macules (ash leaf macules) which are best seen with the aid of Wood's light. The hypopigmented macules are often present at birth, but the facial lesions usually first appear at the age of 5 or 6. Affected individuals may be mentally retarded and suffer from epilepsy. Other features include retinal phakomas, pulmonary and renal harmartomas, and cardiac rhabdomyomas.

Neurofibromatosis

Neurofibromatosis (von Recklinghausen's disease) is a dominantly inherited condition characterized by multiple café-au-lait patches of hyperpigmentation and numerous neurofibromas derived from peripheral nerves (Fig. 11.6). A

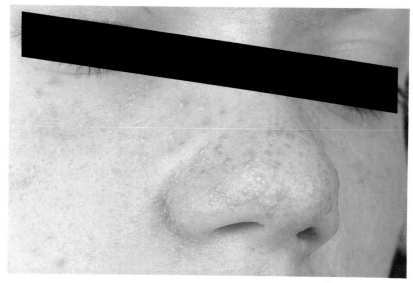

Fig. 11.4. Facial angiofibromas in tuberous sclerosis.

constant feature is the presence of axillary freckling (Crowe's sign). Other associated abnormalities include scoliosis, an increased risk of developing intracranial neoplasms, particularly meningioma, acoustic neuroma and optic nerve glioma, and an increased risk of hypertension associated with phaeochromocytoma or fibromuscular hyperplasia of the renal arteries.

Peutz–Jeghers syndrome

In this rare syndrome pigmented macules (lentigines) are present in the mouth, on the lips, and on the hands and feet, in association with multiple polyps throughout the intestinal tract. The pigmented macules first appear in early childhood, and usually the lesions on the hands and feet regress in adult life. The gut polyps, which are hamartomatous, may cause intussusception. Peutz–Jeghers syndrome is dominantly inherited.

Hereditary haemorrhagic telangiectasia (Osler–Weber–Rondu disease)

This is a rare, dominantly inherited disorder in which multiple telangiectases are present on the face and lips, nasal, buccal and intestinal mucosae. Recurrent epistaxes are the commonest problem in this condition, and there is also a significant risk of gastrointestinal haemorrhage. Attempts to reduce the frequency of epistaxes by treatment with oestrogens, which induce squamous metaplasia of the nasal epithelium, are of limited benefit, and some patients require skin grafting of the nasal septum (septal dermoplasty). There is an association with pulmonary and cerebral arteriovenous fistulae.

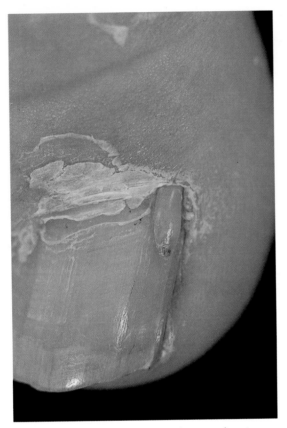

Fig. 11.5. Periungual fibroma in tuberous sclerosis.

Basal cell naevus syndrome (Gorlin's syndrome)

Gorlin's syndrome is a dominantly inherited disorder in which multiple basal cell carcinomas on the face and trunk are associated with characteristic palmar pits, odontogenic keratocysts of the jaw, calcification of the falx cerebri, and skeletal abnormalities.

Gardner's syndrome

This condition is also dominantly inherited. Affected individuals have multiple epidermoid cysts, osteomas, and multiple adenomatous polyps in the large bowel. There is a high risk of malignant change in the gut polyps.

Anhidrotic ectodermal dysplasia

This is a rare condition in which eccrine sweat glands are absent or markedly reduced in number, the scalp hair, eyebrows and eyelashes are sparse, and the teeth are widely spaced and conical in shape. Affected individuals have a characteristic facial appearance. The absence of sweating interferes with temperature regulation and this may lead to hyperthermia in a hot environment. Anhidrotic ectodermal dysplasia is inherited as an X-linked recessive trait.

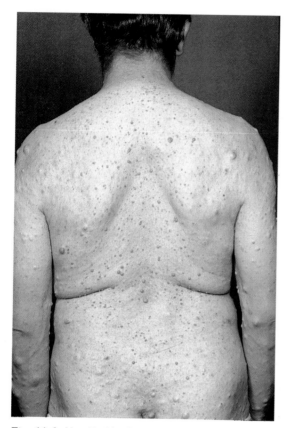

Fig. 11.6. Von Recklinghausen's neurofibromatosis.

Pseudoxanthoma elasticum

Four types, two dominant and two recessive, of this disorder of elastin have been described. Characteristically the skin of the neck and axillae has a lax, 'plucked chicken' appearance of tiny yellowish papules (Fig. 11.7). Retinal angioid streaks, caused by ruptures in the elastin component of Bruch's membrane, are visible on fundoscopy. The elastic tissue of blood vessels is also abnormal, and this may lead to gastrointestinal haemorrhage.

Xeroderma pigmentosum

In normal skin, UV damage to epidermal DNA is repaired by an enzyme system. In xeroderma pigmentosum, which is recessively inherited, this system is defective, and UV damage to the skin is not repaired. This leads to the early development of cutaneous neoplasms in affected individuals. Basal cell carcinomas, squamous cell carcinomas and malignant melanomas may all develop in childhood. In some individuals suffering from xeroderma pigmentosum there is also gradual neurological deterioration caused by progressive neuronal loss.

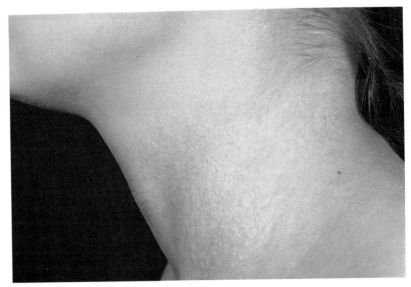

Fig. 11.7. 'Plucked chicken' appearance of the skin in pseudoxanthoma elasticum.

Acrodermatitis enteropathica

In this recessively inherited disorder there is defective absorption of zinc from the gut. The condition usually appears in early infancy with exudative eczematous lesions around the orifices, and on the hands and feet. Affected infants also suffer from diarrhoea. Acrodermatitis enteropathica can be effectively treated with oral zinc supplements.

Anderson–Fabry's disease (angiokeratoma corporis diffusum)

This condition is an inborn error of glycosphingolipid metabolism. It is inherited in an X-linked recessive manner. Deficiency of the enzyme α-galactosidase leads to deposition of ceramide trihexoside in a number of tissues, including the cardiovascular system, the kidneys, the eyes and peripheral nerves. The skin lesions seen in this condition are tiny vascular angiokeratomas which are usually scattered over the lower trunk, buttocks, genitalia and thighs. Associated features caused by tissue deposition of the lipid include premature ischaemic heart disease, renal failure, severe pain and paraesthesiae in the hands and feet, and corneal and lens opacities.

Incontinentia pigmenti

An X-linked dominant disorder, incontinentia pigmenti is seen predominantly in female infants, being usually lethal *in utero* in males. The condition usually presents within a few days of birth as linear bullous lesions on the trunk and limbs. The bullae are gradually replaced over a period of a few weeks by warty lesions, and these in turn are eventually replaced by streaks and whorls of hyperpigmentation. Incontinentia pigmenti is frequently associated with a variety of ocular, skeletal, dental and CNS abnormalities.

Chromosomal abnormalities

Some syndromes associated with chromosomal abnormalities may have associated dermatological problems, for example:

Down's syndrome: increased incidence of alopecia areata

Turner's syndrome: primary lymphoedema

Klinefelter's syndrome: premature venous ulceration

XYY syndrome: premature venous ulceration; prone to develop severe nodulocystic acne

Chapter 12
Pigmentary Disorders

Bold was her face, and fair, and red of hew
(Geoffrey Chaucer,
The Wife of Bath)

The complexion of the skin and the colour of the hair correspond to the colour of the
moisture which the flesh attracts—white, or red, or black
(Hippocrates)

Normal pigmentary mechanisms

Our colour is important to us. This is illustrated by many references to it in prose and poetry throughout the ages: the quote from Chaucer above is but one, early example. Amongst other things, we all take note of another person's skin colour in our initial assessment of them and skin colour has been used, of course, to justify all manner of injustices throughout history. Any departure from the perceived norm can have a serious psychological effect, and may have practical implications as well.

There are a number of factors that give rise to our skin colour: the colour of haemoglobin in circulating blood; the presence of exogenous pigments within or on the surface of the skin; endogenously-produced pigments such as bilirubin. The most important of all in dictating our basic skin colour, however, is the production of melanin and phaeomelanin. The normal pigmentary mechanisms have already been mentioned briefly in Chapter 1. Human beings have a rather dull range of natural colours when compared to, say, a peacock or a parrot. We normally produce only two colours: brown and red. Hippocrates (see above) clearly understood this. The brown colour is created by melanin and the intensity of colour varies from almost white (no melanin) to virtually jet-black (lots of melanin). This is dictated by the individual's genetics in an autosomal dominant manner. Red is a bonus. Only some people can produce the so-called 'phaeomelanin' responsible. It is much commoner in some races (e.g. Celts) than in others (e.g. Chinese).

It is important to understand that most of the pigment in human skin is contained in the keratinocytes, having been manufactured in melanocytes and transferred in packages called melanosomes. There are racial differences in the baseline production, distribution and degradation of melanosomes, but not in the number of melanocytes (see Chapter 1). There are, however, important genetic differences in an individual's ability to respond to UV radiation, conventionally called 'skin types':

Type I: always burns, never tans
Type II: burns easily, tans poorly
Type III: burns occasionally, tans easily
Type IV: never burns, tans easily
Type V: genetically brown (e.g. Indian) or Mongoloid
Type VI: genetically black (Congoid or Negroid)

The early response to UV radiation is an increase in the rate of distribution of melanosomes in those who are able to respond. This produces a rapid increase in basal layer pigmentation—the sun tan. If the stimulation is quickly withdrawn, as typically happens after a brief 2-week bash in the Mediterranean sun, the tan fades rapidly and peels off as normal epidermal turnover continues. If the exposure is more prolonged, melanin production is stepped up on a more permanent basis (again only in those who are capable of the response). This response is an attempt by the skin to offer protection from the more harmful effects of exposure to UV radiation, such as premature ageing and cancers.

We shall now look at states in which these pigmentary mechanisms appear not to be working normally, leading to decreased (hypo-) or increased (hyper-) pigmentation.

Hypopigmentation

There are many causes of hypopigmentation. Among the most important are:
  Congenital:
  Albinism
  Phenylketonuria
  Tuberous sclerosis
  Hypochromic naevi
  Acquired:
  Vitiligo
  Sutton's halo naevi
  Leprosy
  Pityriasis (tinea) versicolor
  Pityriasis alba
  Lichen sclerosus et atrophicus
  Drugs and chemicals: occupational leucoderma; self-inflicted/iatrogenic
  Postinflammatory hypopigmentation

Congenital

Some individuals are born with generalized or localized defects in the pigmentary system leading to hypopigmentation.

Defects in the melanin production pathways occur in *albinism* and *phenylketonuria*. In albinos, the enzyme tyrosinase may be absent (tyrosinase-negative albinism) or defective (tyrosinase-positive albinism.) The result of the former is an individual with generalized white skin and hair. The eyes are red because the iris is also depigmented, and vision is usually markedly reduced, with nystagmus. In tyrosinase-positive albinism, the clinical picture is not usually quite as severe, and the skin and hair may gradually become darker with age. However, skin cancers are much more common in both forms of albinism. Albinism also illustrates how important colour can be: in some societies, albinos are rejected and despised; in others they are revered as something wonderful.

The biochemical defect responsible for phenylketonuria results in reduced amounts of tyrosine, the precursor of melanin, and also raised amounts of phenylalanine which inhibits tyrosinase. This usually produces a generalized reduction in pigmentation of skin, hair and eyes.

One of the cardinal physical signs of *tuberous sclerosis (epiloia)* is the presence of hypopigmented macules. These are often lanceolate in shape (like ash leaves), but may assume more bizarre shapes. These hypopigmented areas are usually present before the other external markers. It is important to examine any infant who presents with fits for such lesions and it may be easier to see them under Wood's light (see Chapter 2) than with the naked eye. Occasionally a child is born without any other features of tuberous sclerosis, but with one or more identical localized pale areas. These are called *hypochromic naevi*.

Acquired

Acquired hypopigmentation is common and can be very distressing. In darker races hypopigmented patches have a particular stigma. This is partly because the background normal skin colour is much darker and the cosmetic appearance of patchy hypopigmentation is much worse. It is also because white patches are inextricably linked in some cultures with leprosy. In past times, too, white patches of all kinds were probably classified as leprosy. It is thought, for example, that Naaman (who was cured of 'leprosy' after bathing in the Jordan) may have had *vitiligo* (2 Kings 5:1–14). The differential diagnosis that needs to be considered when encountering patchy hypopigmentation is listed above.

Vitiligo

This is, perhaps, the most important cause of patches of pale skin. Strictly speaking, the skin in vitiligo is actually *de*pigmented and not hypopigmented, although during *progression* of the process, depigmentation is obviously not always complete.

The characteristic features of an area of vitiligo are of complete loss of pigment from otherwise entirely normal skin (Fig. 12.1). The patches may be small, but it is more common for the areas to become quite large, often with irregular outlines. Occasionally the depigmentation spreads to involve wide areas of the body, resulting in a most unsightly appearance, especially in pigmented skins. Although vitiligo can occur anywhere, it is quite often symmetrical, involving the hands, the perioral and periocular skin.

The cause is unknown, but an autoimmune process seems likely. There is an increased incidence of organ-specific autoantibodies in patients with vitiligo (as in alopecia areata, with which vitiligo is also linked). In early patches of vitiligo the melanocytes are still present, but fail to produce melanin. Later in the course of the disorder, the melanocytes disappear, although they are often still visible in hair follicles.

Treatment is generally unsatisfactory. Topical steroids have their advocates, and PUVA (psoralens + long wave UV radiation) helps some. Cosmetic camouflage may help to hide unsightly areas. Sun screens should be recommended for use in the summer, because vitiliginous areas will not tan.

It is also important to note that in some patients, particularly children, vitiliginous areas may repigment spontaneously. This is a less common

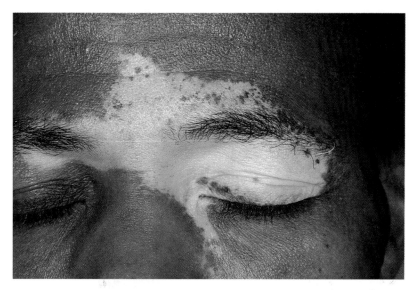

Fig. 12.1. A typical patch of vitiligo.

occurrence in adults and in long-standing areas. Repigmentation, when it does happen, often begins with several small dots of pigment within the patch, coinciding with hair follicles.

A similar appearance to that seen in vitiligo occurs in *Sutton's halo naevus* (*see* Chapter 10).

Some of the stigma associated with hypopigmentation in certain cultures results from the fact that tuberculoid *leprosy* may cause hypopigmentation. In this form of the disease, a solitary patch of hypopigmented skin also exhibits markedly diminished sensation. Pale patches may also be seen in the very earliest stages of the disorder (so-called 'indeterminate' leprosy).

The organism which causes *pityriasis versicolor* (*see* Chapter 4) produces a chemical (azelaic acid) which results in hypopigmentation. The effect is most noticeable after sun exposure.

Pityriasis alba is a very common cause of hypopigmentation in children. It is more prominent in darker skins. Pale patches appear on the face and upper arms (Fig. 12.2). The surface of the patches is slightly scaly. The underlying process is a low-grade eczema and the areas usually respond (albeit slowly) to a moisturiser but sometimes a mild topical steroid is needed. The tendency appears to clear at puberty.

Lichen sclerosus et atrophicus (*see* Chapter 15) is a disorder with a predilection for the genitalia. When it affects other sites it is sometimes called 'white spot disease'.

Drugs and chemicals may cause loss of pigment from the skin. These may be encountered at work, but a more common source is skin lightening creams. These are sold through chemists, especially in areas with high Afro-Caribbean

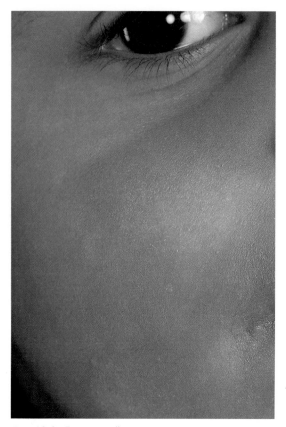

Fig. 12.2. Pityriasis alba.

populations. The active ingredient in most of these is hydroquinone, which can be used therapeutically (see below).

A number of inflammatory skin disorders may produce secondary or *postinflammatory hypopigmentation*. This is extremely common and results from a disturbance in the integrity of the epidermis and its melanin production system. Inflammation may destroy melanocytes altogether. This occurs in scars, after burns and in areas treated with cryotherapy (it is the basis of 'freeze-branding'). Less severe inflammation may disturb the normal distribution of melanosomes temporarily. For example, areas of eczema and psoriasis often leave hypopigmentation behind when they resolve.

Hyperpigmentation

As with hypopigmentation, there are many causes of increased pigmentation in the skin. This may be due to excessive production or collections of melanin, or due to the deposition in the skin of several other pigments, such as β-carotene, bilirubin and drugs and metals:

Congenital

Neurofibromatosis

Peutz–Jegher syndrome
LEOPARD syndrome
Incontinentia pigmenti
Acquired
Urticaria pigmentosa
Addison's disease
Renal failure
Haemochromatosis
Liver disease
Carotenaemia: idiopathic; myxoedema; pernicious anaemia
Acanthosis nigricans
Chloasma
Drugs and chemicals
Postinflammatory hyperpigmentation

Congenital

Hyperpigmentation is an important feature of *neurofibromatosis,* in which café-au-lait marks (Fig. 12.3) and axillary freckling are common. Speckled lentiginous pigmentation is seen around the mouth and on the hands in the *Peutz–Jegher syndrome,* and similar but more widespread lentigines may accompany a number of congenital defects in the so-called *'LEOPARD' syndrome. Incontinentia pigmenti* is another rare congenital disorder which causes hyperpigmentation in a whorled pattern. There may be blisters and hyperkeratotic lesions as well and frequently the child has other congenital abnormalities.

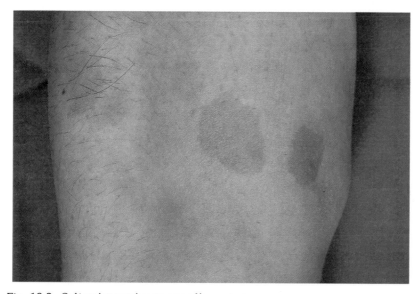

Fig. 12.3. Café-au-lait patches in neurofibromatosis.

Acquired

Urticaria pigmentosa is most commonly seen in children, but it may affect adults. There is a widespread eruption of rather indistinct brown marks which urticate if rubbed. The disorder is due to abnormal accumulations of mast cells in the dermis.

Hyperpigmentation is an important physical sign in a number of systemic diseases. In *Addison's disease* the changes are most marked in the skin creases and in scratch marks, and there may be gum pigmentation. *Renal failure* may cause a muddy brown skin colour. Patients with *haemochromatosis* develop a deep golden brown hue, in addition to diabetes and liver disease. Some patients with *liver disease* become deeply pigmented. This may be due to bilirubin, but hypermelanosis also occurs in some liver diseases, especially primary biliary cirrhosis.

Beta-carotene, a yellow pigment, may accumulate in the skin in some apparently normal individuals who simply eat a large amount in their daily diet. Carrots and orange juice are rich sources. The colour is most marked on the palms and soles. Carotenaemia does no harm. Similar deposition occurs in

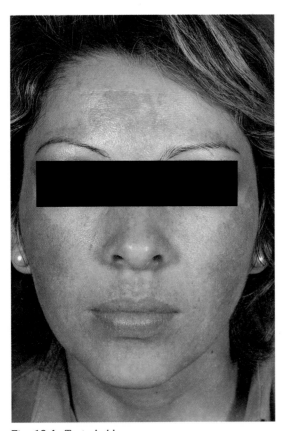

Fig. 12.4. Typical chloasma.

some patients with myxoedema and pernicious anaemia, in whom a 'lemon-yellow' skin tint is an important physical sign.

Another cause of acquired hyperpigmentation is *acanthosis nigricans*. This may or may not be associated with a systemic disease (see Chapter 19).

Chloasma, or melasma, is a common presenting symptom. It is much commoner in women. A characteristic pattern of hyperpigmentation develops on the forehead, cheeks and chin (Fig. 12.4). It is exaggerated by sunlight. Chloasma may be provoked by pregnancy or the oral contraceptive pill, but it may also occur spontaneously. Treatment is difficult. Avoidance of precipitating factors such as sunlight and exogenous oestrogens may help. Topical hydroquinone preparations are sometimes used.

Various *drugs and chemicals* can cause cutaneous hyperpigmentation (see Chapter 21).

In *postinflammatory hyperpigmentation* disruption of the lower layers of the epidermis results in deposition of melanin granules in the underlying dermis (pigmentary incontinence). Many skin disorders may do this, particularly in pigmented skin. Lichen planus is particularly prone to leave this kind of pigmentary abnormality. There is no useful treatment but the areas will gradually fade with time.

Chapter 13
Disorders of the Hair and Nails

If a woman have long hair, it is a glory to her.
(1 Cor.11:15)

The hair takes root in the head at the same time as the nails grow.
(Hippocrates)

Abnormalities of the hair and nails may be the result of local factors, generalized skin diseases or systemic disease. In this chapter we shall look at the most important hair and nail changes that will be seen in clinical practice. As implied by the quote from Hippocrates above, disease processes may affect both hair and nails at the same time but there are also many conditions which affect one or the other independently. In this chapter we will deal first with abnormalities of hair and then with nail disorders, but there will be some overlap between the two.

Hair abnormalities

Hair is very important psychologically and disturbances in its growth or physical characteristics, even of quite minor degree, may be very distressing: only Kojak really likes being bald. As with other skin complaints, the apparent distress suffered does not necessarily relate to the absolute severity of the problem. Patients present for medical advice with three main abnormalities of their hair: a change in the physical property of the hair, such as its texture or colour, thinning or loss of hair, and excessive hair growth, including the growth of hair in abnormal sites. Most of the clinical problems of the first two relate to scalp hair, although hair loss may occur occasionally from other sites.

Changes in physical properties of scalp hair

Common physical changes that are seen in hair include:
Pigmentation
    Genetic diseases, e.g. albinism, phenylketonuria
    Premature greying: physiological; pathological, e.g. pernicious anaemia
    Ageing
    Vitiligo
    Alopecia areata
Textural abnormalities
    Brittleness
    Coarseness
    Curliness

Change in colour

There is, of course, very little that can be done about canities or greying of the hair, whether it is premature or not, apart from dyeing it. There are many dyes available, some of which cause contact dermatitis. The white hair seen in vitiligo of the scalp is often also permanent, especially in adults. Hair regrowing in areas of alopecia areata are often white initially, but usually return to their normal colour (see below).

Textural abnormalities

Brittleness or coarseness of the hair may accompany hair thinning in hypothyroidism and in iron deficiency (see below). Hair may also become coarse and 'lack-lustre' from constant use of certain hairdressing techniques, such as back-combing, bleaching and drying with hot air. In men, hair may become curly in areas affected by the early stages of androgenetic alopecia (see below).

Scalp hair loss

Congenital disorders

There are a number of rare disorders in which abnormal scalp hair growth is one of the important features: ectodermal dysplasias, premature ageing syndromes. There are also congenital conditions in which hair abnormalities are the main or the only complaint: monilethrix, pili torti, Marie–Unna alopecia, disorders of amino acid metabolism. Most of these conditions are not amenable to treatment. They require careful assessment, often including microscopic examination of hair shafts. Naevi of the scalp (especially epithelial and organoid types) may also lead to an area of alopecia. Localized hair loss on the scalp at birth may be due to a developmental failure: aplasia cutis.

Acquired disorders

Although there are, of course, several hair bearing sites the most common reason for a patient to seek medical advice is when there is loss of scalp hair. The traditional (and still the most effective) way of approaching the diagnosis of acquired scalp hair loss is to consider whether the changes are diffuse or circumscribed and also to assess the state of the scalp skin. Such an approach, together with the most important causes (elaborated below) leads to the classification given in Table 13.1. The first step in diagnosing acquired scalp hair loss, therefore, is to establish the pattern and to determine whether or not there is any obvious abnormality of the scalp.

Diffuse hair loss with normal scalp skin

The most important causes of diffuse hair loss with no scalp changes are: telogen effluvium; endocrine disease; iron deficiency; drugs; and androgenetic alopecia. Alopecia totalis may also produce this picture.

Telogen effluvium is a well-recognized phenomenon often triggered by a major illness, operation, accident or other stressful event. This results in a sudden cessation of growth of a large number of hairs which rapidly enter the resting or telogen phase. These hairs begin to fall out in large numbers about 3 months later (the normal daily hair loss of telogen hairs is about 100). It is

Table 13.1. Scalp hair loss

Diffuse hair loss with normal scalp skin
Telogen effluvium
Thyroid disease
Iron deficiency
Drugs
Systemic lupus erythematosus
Alopecia totalis
Secondary syphilis

Androgenetic alopecia

Circumscribed hair loss with normal scalp skin
Alopecia areata
Traction
Trichotillomania
Tinea capitis (Chapter 4)

Hair loss with abnormal scalp skin
Without scarring
  Severe psoriasis or seborrhoeic dermatitis
  Tinea capitis (chapter 4)
With scarring
  Discoid lupus erythematosus
  Lichen planus
  Pseudopelade
  Cicatricial pemphigoid
  Trigeminal trophic syndrome
  Lupus vulgaris
  Tinea capitis (Chapter 4)

---

important, therefore to ask specifically whether any such major upset has occurred over the appropriate period. It may be helpful to pull gently on the hairs on the crown or sides of the head. In a telogen effluvium several hairs will come out without much effort and the bulb can be seen under a hand lens to be much smaller than a normal, growing hair. A telogen effluvium usually settles spontaneously but it can unmask an underlying androgenetic alopecia (see below) and some patients find that their scalp hair never really returns completely to normal.

It is always important in any patient with diffuse hair loss to look for signs of *myxoedema or thyrotoxicosis* and to check for *iron deficiency*. Correction of these may restore normal hair growth. It is also essential that a good drug history be taken. There are many drugs that can induce hair loss in addition to the cytotoxic agents (where it is often an expected side-effect): antithyroid agents, especially thiouracil; anticoagulants; the new vitamin A analogues etretinate and isotretinoin; and thallium. Both *systemic lupus erythematosus* and *secondary syphilis* may also give rise to hair loss. This is often rather patchy, leaving a 'moth-eaten' appearance. This can be confused with widespread alopecia areata (see below).

Androgenetic alopecia (common balding) occurs in both men and women. It is thought to be due to the effects of androgens in genetically susceptible individuals.

In men, the process may begin at any age after puberty, but it is much more common from the 30s onwards. By the eighth decade about 80% of men show some hair loss of this kind. Hair is lost first at the temples and/or on the crown, but the ultimate result may be complete hair loss, sparing a parieto-occipital rim. The terminal hairs become progressively finer and smaller, until all that remains are a few vellus hairs. The extent and pace of this process varies widely.

In women the process is usually slower and less severe than in men but it still causes much distress. In fact, up to half of all women have some frontal loss by the age of 50 but in some, especially as they pass into the 60s and beyond, a more severe degree of thinning occurs, which is most marked on the vertex. The hair density decreases and the remaining hair becomes much finer. There may be accompanying hirsutism (see below), but this is by no means always the case.

Until recently there was no known treatment for this type of hair loss. However, topical minoxidil may arrest the process, if it is used early enough.

Alopecia totalis, a severe form of alopecia areata (see below), may present with diffuse hair loss.

Circumscribed hair loss with normal scalp skin

By far the commonest and most important cause of circumscribed hair loss with apparently normal scalp skin is *alopecia areata*. In this condition one or more areas of complete baldness suddenly appear. These may occur anywhere on the scalp, in the eyebrows, beard, or indeed elsewhere. The process most commonly begins in childhood or early adult life, although periodic recurrences throughout life may occur and it can begin much later.

The patches are often round or oval in shape (Fig. 13.1) and the skin usually appears completely normal, although there may be mild erythema. Sometimes a number of small areas may develop in close proximity to each other, giving rise to a moth-eaten appearance. Close examination of the edge of a patch of alopecia areata reveals the presence of short hairs which seem to taper towards their base (Fig. 13.2). These are called 'exclamation mark hairs' and are pathognomonic of the disorder.

In most patients the patches regrow after a few weeks, although further episodes may continue to occur. The initial hair growth is quite often white. Occasionally, the process continues to spread and may become permanent. If this state involves the whole scalp it is termed *alopecia totalis*. If the whole body is affected, the name *alopecia universalis* is applied. The nails may be affected in severe cases (see below).

The cause of this disorder is unknown but it is strongly suspected that it is an autoimmune process. Organ-specific autoantibodies (to thyroid, adrenal or gastric parietal cell) are often found in the patients' serum. Treatment is difficult, but intralesional steroids have some effect in promoting new growth, and topical

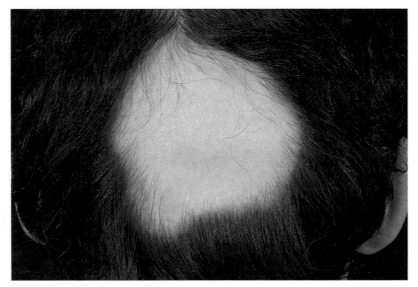

Fig. 13.1. A typical patch of alopecia areata.

sensitizers such as dinitrochlorobenzene and diphencyprone also appear to promote growth in some patients by inducing a contact dermatitis.

Chronic traction can also cause circumscribed alopecia. For example, it is quite common for young girls to wear their hair in a tight 'pony tail', and this may lead to loss around the frontal scalp margins (Fig. 13.3). Sikh boys may

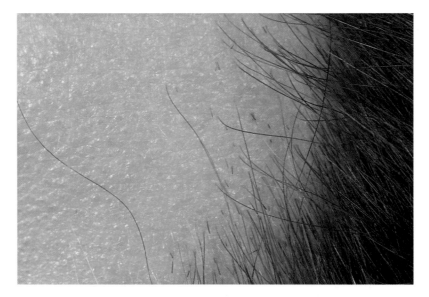

Fig. 13.2. The edge of the area seen in Fig. 13.1. Exclamation mark hairs are visible at the margin.

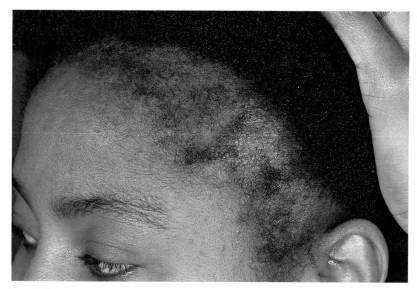

Fig. 13.3. Traction alopecia.

develop this too, as may Afro-Caribbean children whose hair is dressed in multiple little 'pigtails'.

Another condition which may give rise to this problem is *trichotillomania,* where the hair is literally pulled, twisted or rubbed out. This usually occurs in childhood and is associated with psychological, behavioural and learning problems. The affected site(s) are covered in stubble with broken hairs. The child often seems relatively unperturbed.

Hair loss with abnormal scalp skin

Any inflammatory process in the scalp, such as psoriasis or seborrhoeic dermatitis, can give rise to temporary hair loss. By far the commonest cause of temporary hair loss with scalp inflammation is tinea capitis (see Chapter 4). In these situations, regrowth generally occurs after the inflammation has settled.

However, in some disease states the process results in permanent damage to hair follicles. Fibrosis often accompanies such changes and this leads to a clinical appearance of obvious loss of tissue or atrophy. Such a state is known as a scarring or cicatricial alopecia.

The most important causes of cicatricial alopecia are listed above. It is important to look for specific signs of each of these conditions, including at other sites. In *discoid lupus erythematosus* there may be prominent plugging of the hair follicles in the patches themselves, but the presence of lesions on the face would be of more diagnostic importance. *Lichen planus* of the scalp may accompany lichen planus on the skin or in the mouth, but nail involvement is especially important. This may be gross or consist of quite subtle ridging and linear depressions. Either of these two conditions may also give rise to *pseudopelade,* a clinical appearance of small patches of scarring alopecia with no other distinguishing features. Occasionally, such an appearance may arise quite independently. In *cicatricial pemphigoid* a scarring alopecia follows blistering. *Lupus vulgaris* (cutaneous tuberculosis) should not be forgotten, especially in a patient who has lived in an endemic area such as India. *Trigeminal trophic syndrome* may follow herpes zoster with or without a subsequent nerve block for trigeminal neuralgia. The resulting hypoaesthesia allows chronic damage to the scalp to occur without the patient noticing, and a circumscribed patch of hair loss is not uncommon.

In most of the conditions described above, a biopsy is essential in making the correct diagnosis. In cases where lupus erythematosus or cicatricial pemphigoid are suspected, immunofluorescence should also be performed.

Generalized hair loss

Generalized hair loss is rare. It may accompany endocrine disturbances, especially *hypothyroidism* or *hypopituitarism*. *Drugs,* particularly cytotoxics may induce widespread alopecia. As has already been mentioned, the disease state we call alopecia areata may lead to complete hair loss—*alopecia universalis.*

Excessive hair and hair in abnormal sites

When excessive hair growth is the main complaint, it is important first to distinguish between *hirsutism* and *hypertrichosis*. The term *hirsutism* should be reserved for excessive growth of hair in a female which is distributed in a male secondary sexual pattern. This occurs fairly frequently in elderly women who often develop moustaches and beards. It is also seen as a genetic trait, passed on from mother to daughter. Hirsutism may accompany a general reduction in scalp hair (see androgenetic alopecia above). Although most instances fall into one of these three categories, it is also important to remember that drugs with androgenic activity and virilizing tumours may induce hirsutism. A search for such a cause should certainly be undertaken if the changes are of rapid onset.

Treatment is usually destructive: shaving; waxing; or electrolysis. The antiandrogen cyproterone acetate may help.

Hypertrichosis or excessive hair growth in a non-sexual distribution may occur in both sexes. There are a few rare congenital causes of generalized hypertrichosis such as the Cornelia de Lange syndrome. Localized overgrowth of hair on the lower back (faun-tail) may be a sign of underlying spinal defects.

Drugs such as minoxidil (now a recognized treatment for baldness—see above) and cyclosporin A are two of the newer agents which promote hair growth but hydantoins, systemic steroids and others have long been known to be responsible. Hypertrichosis also occurs in association with scarring and milia on the face in porphyria cutanea tarda and may be seen overlying plaques of pretibial myxoedema in a patient with Graves' disease. A generalized overproduction of fine, lanugo hairs is occasionally seen in patients with an underlying cancer or with cachexia whatever the cause.

Nail abnormalities

A number of changes in the nails may bring them to the attention of the patient and, subsequently, the doctor.

The nails are abnormal in some *congenital disorders*. This is particularly true of conditions in which there are primary defects in the processes of keratinization or of the production of the epidermis as a whole, such as ectodermal dysplasias and Darier's disease (see Chapter 11). Nails may also be damaged or even lost altogether in some congenital disorders, due to scarring secondary to the primary disease process. A good example of this is dystrophic epidermolysis bullosa (Chapter 14).

There are many *acquired nail abnormalities*. Some changes are relatively disease-specific: the nails are often affected in some common skin diseases:

1 Psoriasis (see Chapter 8).
2 Eczema/dermatitis (see Chapter 7).
3 Lichen planus (see Chapter 15).
4 Alopecia areata/totalis: see below.
5 Fungal infections (see Chapter 4).

Other nail changes are more non-specific reflections of an alteration in nail growth and may occur for no apparent reason. However, sometimes nail dystrophies represent a more generalized disturbance.

Brittleness is a common complaint. There is an increasing tendency for the nail plate to crack easily with increasing age, but it may also occur as a result of iron deficiency (see also koilonychia) and thyroid deficiency.

Roughness of the nails (or trachyonchia) is also a fairly common and rather non-specific symptom. Occasionally, very bad pitting (see below) results in a rough nail surface.

Beau's lines is the name given to horizontal grooves which appear in the nails, usually after a major illness.

Pits in the nails are one of the classical features of psoriasis but they may also be seen in severe alopecia areata/totalis when they are usually smaller and more evenly distributed than in psoriasis, and affect all the nails. Dents and pits are also seen in the nails of fingers which are badly affected by eczema.

Onycholysis means lifting of the nail plate away from the nail bed. There are several causes:

1 Psoriasis.
2 Onycholysis may occur in the absence of any other identifiable abnormality (Fig. 13.4).
3 Fungal nail infection (see Chapter 4).
4 Thyrotoxicosis.

The nail plate may also be lifted up by a space-occupying lesion, such as a tumour or an exostosis of the underlying distal phalanx.

Clubbing is a well-known sign of internal disease, especially pulmonary or thyroid. It may also occur as a familial trait. *Discoloration* of the nail plate may be due to several different conditions. *Horizontal white marks* are an extremely common normal variant, but if the whole nail plate is white, there may be underlying cirrhosis. Fungal infections generally cause the nail plate to be a

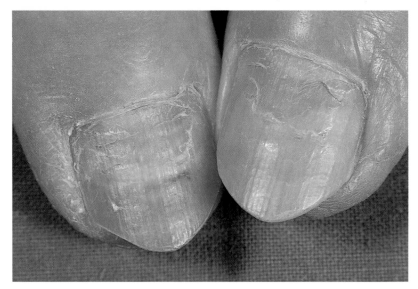

Fig. 13.4. Onycholysis of the nails in a woman with no other relevant findings.

patchy *sulphur-yellow* colour. Uniformly yellow nails occur in a rare disorder called the yellow nail syndrome, in which patients may also develop bronchiectasis and lymphoedema. Pseudomonas infection of the nail bed gives a *greeny blue* patch under the nail. The nails are *pale* in anaemia, and *half pale, half red-brown* in severe renal disease ('half-and-half nails'). *Brown or black* areas under the nail may be due to altered blood, a pigmented naevus or a malignant melanoma. On the fingers, there is usually a clear history of preceding injury if the lesion is a haematoma. However, on the toes subungual collections of blood are quite common without any clear history of trauma being elicited. Another common feature are pigmented linear bands in the nails. These are usually due to naevi in the nail fold. Melanomas cause irregular areas of dark pigmentation, often involving the nail fold (see Chapter 9).

  Koilonychia is the termed used to describe nails with a concave upper surface, giving rise to a spoon shape. The most important association with this is iron deficiency, although koilonychia may also be inherited.

  When nail damage is severe, the surrounding epithelium may begin to encroach on to the surface of what was once the nail plate. This is called *pterygium*, and is most common in severe lichen planus of the nail apparatus (Chapter 15). Ultimately, and if unchecked, pterygium will lead to *complete distortion and destruction* of the nails. Other disease processes which lead to scarring, such as the Stevens–Johnson syndrome, may also cause complete loss of nails. Very severe inflammation alone can also produce virtual destruction of the normal nail architecture. A good example of this is pustular psoriasis (see Chapter 8). Malignant melanomas or squamous cell carcinomas also destroy the nail, and should be considered if there is only one affected digit.

Washboard nails are a relatively common abnormality which is due to repeated rubbing of the nail fold in a habit-tic.

Onychogryphosis is a state in which the nails become grossly thickened and distorted (Fig. 13.5). It may follow trauma to the nail, but is also a common finding in tramps and others who are not overscrupulous about their feet, suggesting that poorly fitting shoes and hygiene may be important factors.

Common disorders of the paronychium

Patients may also complain of disorders of the area around the nail (the paronychium):

Paronychia

There are two common forms of paronychia: acute and chronic. In acute paronychia, there is an abscess in the nail fold. This eventually points and discharges. It is nearly always staphylococcal. Chronic paronychia is discussed in Chapter 4.

Ingrowing nails

overcurved nails, especially on the big toes, tend to dig into the lateral nail fold and create a chronic inflammatory reaction with an overproduction of granulation tissue. The best treatment is prevention, by trimming the nails straight across. However, surgical intervention may be required if the process is too painful.

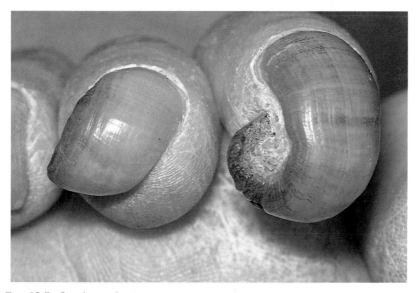

Fig. 13.5. Onychogryphosis.

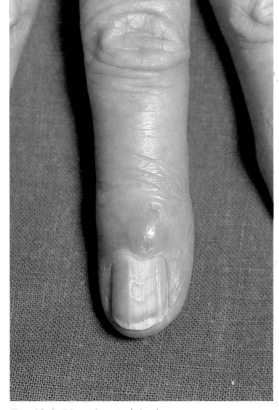

Fig. 13.6. Myxoid cyst of the finger.

Periungual warts

Warts are discussed in Chapter 3. Periungual warts can be very unsightly and are often extremely difficult to eradicate.

Myxoid cyst

This is a common lesion in the middle-aged and elderly. A small cystic swelling develops near the proximal nail fold (Fig. 13.6). The nail may grow out with a linear depression. If the surface of the cyst is breached, a clear gelatinous fluid can be expressed. Treatment is difficult.

Chapter 14
Bullous Disorders

All that blisters is not pemphigus

The skin has a limited repertoire of changes, but there are few more dramatic than an eruption of blisters or bullae. There are many causes (Table 14.1): this table provides a fairly comprehensive differential diagnostic list for further reading, and it would be nice to deal with each of the entities mentioned above in detail but this is not appropriate for a book of this size. Some, such as impetigo and the viral causes, are covered elsewhere, and this chapter is concerned with the most important of the remaining causes of blistering.

Physical causes of bullae

Burns, whether cold, heat or chemical are well-known and frequently encountered causes. Extreme friction may also produce blisters. An example of this is the feet of vigorous squash players or joggers. Severe, acute oedema, generally of the lower legs in congestive cardiac failure may give rise to large, tense bullae.

Arthropods

Although dealt with in Chapter 5, it is worth emphasizing here that insect bites on the lower legs very commonly present as tense bullae. In the United Kingdom, this is most commonly seen in girls in the late summer and early autumn (fall).

Drugs

Several drugs are associated with blistering. Those caused by nalidixic acid occur on the lower legs following sun exposure. Fixed drug eruptions may blister and are discussed in Chapter 21.

Skin disorders

Primary skin disorders giving rise to bullae may be congenital or acquired. In some of the acquired conditions, the bullae are an important or integral part of the clinical presentation. In others bulla formation may occur but this is not the most prominent or constant feature. The reader is referred to the appropriate chapter of the book for further information on this group.

Congenital

Epidermolysis bullosa

This is a very rare group of disorders in which babies are born with fragile skin which blisters on contact. This is due to a split within the skin which may occur at different levels. There are several variants:

Table 14.1. Causes of blisters or bullae

Physical
  Cold; heat; friction; oedema

Infections (see Chapter 3,4)
  Bacterial
    Impetigo
  Viral
    Chicken pox
    Herpes zoster
    Herpes simplex
    Smallpox and vaccinia
    Hand, foot and mouth disease
  Fungal
    Tinea pedis with pompholyx

Arthropods (see Chapter 5)
  Insect bites

Drugs (see also Chapter 21)
  Barbiturates; sulphonamides; iodides; frusemide
  Nalidixic acid (light induced)
  Drug-induced pemphigus and pemphigoid
  Fixed drug eruptions

Skin disorders
  Congenital
    Epidermolysis bullosa
  Acquired
    Bullae are a major feature:
      Pemphigus
      Bullous pemphigoid
      Cicatricial pemphigoid
      Dermatitis herpetiformis
      'Linear IgA disease'
      Epidermolysis bullosa acquisita
      Toxic epidermal necrolysis
    Bullae may occur:
      Erythema multiforme (Stevens–Johnson syndrome)
      Eczema (including pompholyx)
      Lichen planus
      Vasculitis

Metabolic disease
  Porphyria cutanea tarda; diabetes mellitus

---

1 *Epidermolysis bullosa simplex* Blisters occur on sites of friction, but heal without scarring and there are few serious sequelae. One variant affects only the hands and feet.
2 *Dystrophic epidermolysis bullosa* In the recessively inherited form of this nasty disease, mutilating scarring of the hands and feet may occur.

3 *Junctional epidermolysis bullosa* (The term 'junctional' refers to the level of the split at which blistering occurs.) Severe forms of junctional epidermolysis bullosa (also known as Herlitz disease) are incompatible with survival beyond the first few months of life.

The diagnosis of these disorders rests on good biopsies for electron microscopic examination (largely to determine the level of the blister). However, the differential diagnosis of blistering in a neonate must include a number of other disorders including impetigo (pemphigus neonatorum), staphylococcal scalded skin syndrome (see below) and incontinentia pigmenti (Chapter 11).

Acquired

Pemphigus

The cardinal process in all forms of pemphigus is a split within the epidermis together with a loss of adhesion of epidermal cells, known as 'acantholysis'. This may occur just above the basal layer or higher in the epidermis. This variation is reflected in the clinical expression of the disease which is classified conventionally into pemphigus vulgaris, pemphigus vegetans, pemphigus foliaceous and pemphigus erythematosus.

Pemphigus vulgaris is the commonest form of pemphigus. The split is just above the basal layer (Fig. 14.1). It presents with flaccid blisters and erosions (Fig. 14.2). These may be anywhere on the body surface but in more than 50% of patients the disorder begins in the mouth, and lesions in the perineum are also common. The blisters rupture easily and the underlying eroded area usually heals very slowly, if at all. This often results in large, non-healing erosions, similar to burns. A highly characteristic feature is the Nikolsky sign: the skin adjacent to a blister slides off when pushed by a finger or when the edge of an erosion is picked up with forceps. This sign is virtually pathognomonic of pemphigus, being seen only in this disorder and in toxic epidermal necrolysis (see below). In the mouth it is unusual to see anything other than erosions (Fig. 14.3), which may be very extensive. Pemphigus vegetans is a variant of

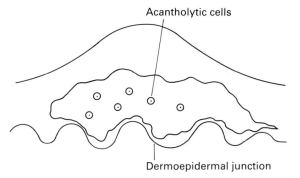

Acantholytic cells

Dermoepidermal junction

Fig. 14.1. Pemphigus vulgaris: split just above the basal layer with overlying acantholysis of epidermal cells.

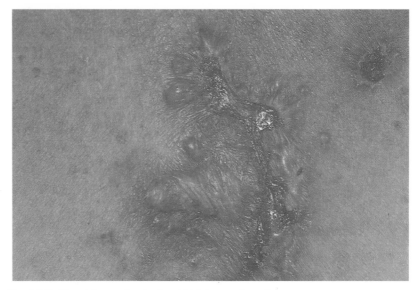

Fig. 14.2. Pemphigus vulgaris: flaccid blisters and erosions.

pemphigus vulgaris in which bulla formation is obscured by large vegetating masses, most commonly occurring in the flexures and in and around the mouth.

In pemphigus foliaceous and erythematosus the cleft is high in the epidermis (Fig. 14.4). This results in several clinical differences. Blisters are even more fragile and are, as a consequence, less apparent than in pemphigus vulgaris. In the earlier stages, there are often rather non-specific scaly areas. The process may begin on the head and face and can closely simulate severe seborrhoeic

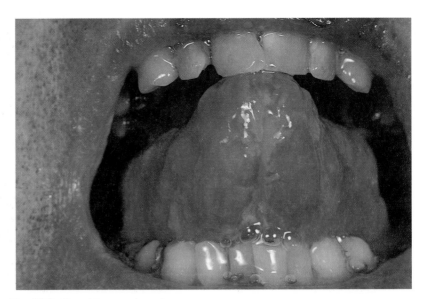

Fig. 14.3. Pemphigus: oral erosions.

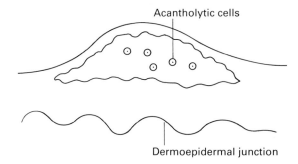

Acantholytic cells

Dermoepidermal junction

Fig. 14.4. Pemphigus foliaceous: similar changes to Fig. 14.1 but higher in the epidermis.

eczema. The variant known as pemphigus erythematosus remains localized to the face, resulting in a scaly rash which may be confused with lupus erythematosus.

The investigations required and subsequent management of all forms of pemphigus are the same. Biopsies should be taken from involved skin, preserving a blister intact if at all possible, and sent for histopathology. Perilesional tissue should be submitted to direct immunofluorescence and serum should always be sent for indirect immunofluorescence as well.

The immunopathology of pemphigus vulgaris, vegetans and foliaceous is identical. There is bright staining around epidermal cells with antibodies directed against IgG and C3 (Fig. 14.5). There is also a circulating anti-epithelial antibody in the majority of patients. In pemphigus erythematosus, a linear band of IgM is also seen at the basement membrane zone.

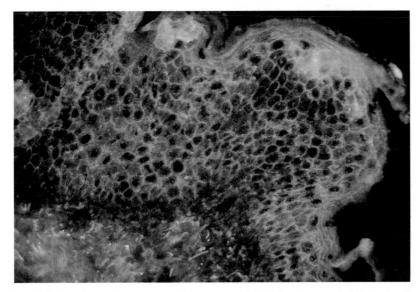

Fig. 14.5. Pemhigus: direct immunofluorescence. IgG is found around epidermal cells.

The treatment of pemphigus needs to be vigorous. Before the advent of systemic corticosteroids most patients died of the disease, often after a long and debilitating illness. High doses of prednisolone (60–120 mg a day) are used, followed by a gradual reduction once new blistering has ceased, which is usually in about 4–6 weeks. Another immunosuppressive agent such as azathioprine, chlorambucil, cyclophosphamide or methotrexate is usually added as a steroid-sparing agent.

Pemphigus often results in a marked systemic disturbance. The patient is unwell and the presence of widespread erosions act like widespread burns, with loss of protein and fluid. There is a marked risk of secondary infection. If the mouth is severely involved, patients often have difficulty in maintaining an adequate calorie and protein intake and may be severely catabolic. Good general nursing and metabolic management are therefore also important.

Finally, it is worth mentioning that pemphigus has been reported in association with a variety of different neoplasms and other disorders, especially myasthenia gravis, and that it may result from drug therapy. The most notable cause is D-penicillamine.

Bullous pemphigoid and cicatricial pemphigoid

Bullous pemphigoid is not all that rare. It is much more common in the elderly, more than 80% of patients being over 60 years of age at presentation.

Although bullae are the most important feature of bullous pemphigoid, they are not always present initially. The process may begin with a rather non-specific phase known as pre-pemphigoid. This is characterized by intense irritation followed by well-defined, slightly elevated, erythematous areas. The bullae, when they do develop, are tense, dome-shaped and multiple (Fig. 14.6). They

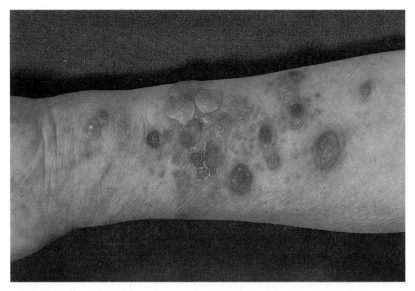

Fig. 14.6. Bullous pemphigoid: tense blisters with an erythematous base arising on a typical site.

may be blood-filled. They vary in size from a few millimetres to several centimetres in diameter. They often arise on areas of urticated erythema as described above, but they are also seen on apparently normal skin. Although the lesions may appear anywhere on the body surface, there is a marked predilection for the limbs. The mouth may be involved in about 30% of patients.

When the blisters burst healing is rapid in most instances although there is a risk of secondary infection which may delay this. Many blisters, however, do not burst and the fluid contents are simply resorbed. The lesions in bullous pemphigoid normally heal without scarring, but there is a distinctive variant in which marked scarring results. This is known as cicatricial or benign mucous membrane pemphigoid.

This is much rarer but is also seen predominantly in the elderly. There are two clinical features that distinguish between cicatricial and bullous pemphigoid: the occurrence of scarring in cicatricial pemphigoid, and the marked predilection of cicatricial pemphigoid for involvement of oral, conjunctival and genital epithelium. The blisters heal to leave depressed, atrophic scars. Scarring also occurs in the mouth and may extend into the pharynx and larynx. Penile and vulval lesions may leave permanent stenoses. The most troublesome complication is the scarring that occurs in the eyes, which may result in adhesion between adjacent conjunctival surfaces, leading to symblepharon. Ultimately this may lead to blindness.

The diagnosis in bullous and cicatricial pemphigoid can be confirmed by a biopsy for histopathology and a biopsy and serum for immunopathology. Histology in both shows a subepidermal blister (Fig. 14.7). Direct immunofluorescence shows a linear band of IgG and C3 at the basement membrane zone (Fig. 14.8). Blood should also be taken for indirect immunofluorescence because 70% of patients with bullous pemphigoid have a circulating IgG class antibody to basement membrane. There is seldom a demonstrable circulating antibody present in cicatricial pemphigoid.

Both pemphigoid variants require treatment with systemic steroids, in moderately high doses initially, and immunosuppressives such as azathioprine or chlorambucil. In bullous pemphigoid, the process usually responds rapidly, and doses can be reduced. Since bullous pemphigoid appears to be self-limiting, it is often possible eventually to cease all treatment. However, it may take up to 5 years to do this. Cicatricial pemphigoid is much less responsive.

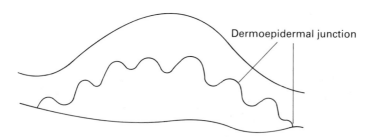

Dermoepidermal junction

Fig. 14.7. Bullous pemphigoid: the split is subepidermal.

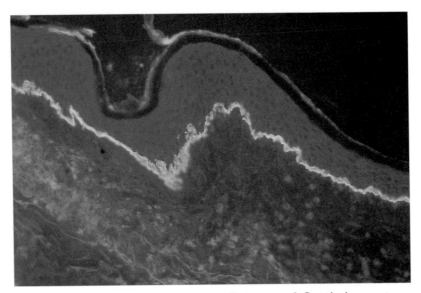

Fig. 14.8. Bullous pemphigoid: direct immunofluorescence. IgG at the basement membrane zone.

There have been many suggestions that bullous pemphigoid may be related to an underlying cancer in some patients, but this remains controversial.

Dermatitis herpetiformis and 'linear IgA disease'

Dermatitis herpetiformis is a rare disorder. However, it is a condition which can remain undiagnosed for many years and seldom undergoes spontaneous remission. Its importance lies in its ability to cause distressing chronic itching, and in its association with a gluten-sensitive enteropathy.

Clinically, the disease is characterized by pruritus. Indeed, if it is thought of exclusively as a 'bullous' disease, it will be missed more often that it is diagnosed. The classical features are of grouped erythematous papules, with occasional vesicles visible, most frequently located on the elbows (Fig. 14.9) and extensor surface of the forearms, knees and shins, buttocks and sometimes the shoulders and scalp. The effects of scratching are usually prominent with excoriations, secondary eczematization and even lichenification. It is often difficult to find vesicles or bullae because of the scratching. The condition should therefore be considered whenever atypical eczema or pruritus is localized to the areas mentioned above.

Histopathologically, the condition shows a subepidermal blister indistinguishable, when fully formed and intact, from that seen in bullous pemphigoid. However, in very early, prevesicular lesions and at the edge of a developing blister, there are small aggregations of neutrophil polymorphonuclear leucocytes in the dermal papillary tips (Fig. 14.10). These so-called 'microabscesses' are pathognomonic of the disorder.

As with pemphigoid and pemphigus, it is also valuable to send skin for immunopathological examination. However, in dermatitis herpetiformis the

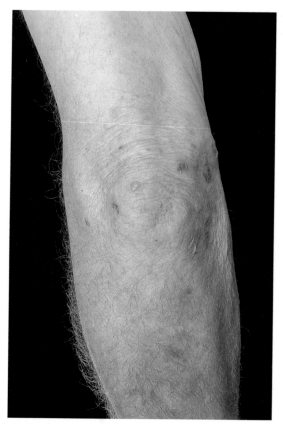

Fig. 14.9. Dermatitis herpetiformis: the elbow is a typical site.

skin sample should be taken from completely normal skin, usually from a covered area such as the buttock or lower back. The diagnostic finding is of granular IgA in the dermal papillary tips (Fig. 14.11). There are no circulating antibodies. It has also long been recognized that IgA may be deposited in the skin as a linear basement membrane zone band (similar in pattern to that seen

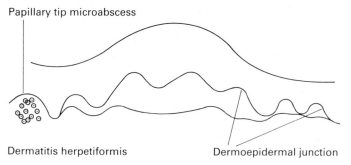

Fig. 14.10. Dermatitis herpetiformis: papillary tip microabscesses as well as a subepidermal blister.

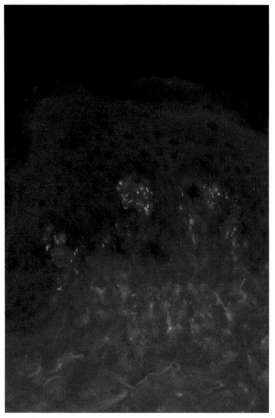

Fig. 14.11. Dermatitis herpetiformis: immunofluorescence of normal skin. Granular deposits of IgA in dermal papillae.

with IgG in Fig. 14.8) and there has been some controversy as to what this represents. Originally, it was classified simply as a variant of dermatitis herpetiformis. More recently, it has been suggested that the pattern of linear IgA represents the immunological marker of a separate bullous disease, labelled 'linear IgA disease'. This pattern is also seen in a rare blistering disorder of childhood known as chronic bullous disorder of childhood. Indeed these conditions may be one and the same.

Dermatitis herpetiformis is frequently associated with a gluten-sensitive enteropathy, which can be demonstrated on jejunal biopsy. This is of considerable importance, since it is claimed that gluten avoidance alone may control the skin lesions and because there may be an increased risk of gut lymphomas, similar to coeliac disease.

Treatment of dermatitis herpetiformis relies on the condition's dramatic responsiveness to sulphones. Dapsone is the drug of choice in most cases and is nearly always dramatically effective. Its use, however, is governed by its side-effects. It induces haemolysis, especially at higher doses, and can precipitate a marked drop in haemoglobin. Alternatives that can be used are sulphapyridine and sulphamethoxypyridazine. Patients in whom a gluten-sensitivity has been demonstrated should also be started on a gluten-free diet.

Rarer blistering diseases

Porphyria cutanea tarda

This is a very rare disorder. Although familial cases have now been reported in whom the disease may present early in life, in the majority of patients symptoms and signs occur for the first time in the fourth or fifth decades or beyond. The characteristic early cutaneous features are small blisters and erosions on the backs of the hands, the forearms and the face following minor trauma. The areas heal to leave scarring and milia formation. Later there may be marked hyperpigmentation, hypertrichosis and pseudosclerodermatous thickening of the skin. Similar changes are seen in variegate porphyria, a disorder almost unique to families of Dutch or South African descent, and in some patients with chronic renal failure, when the condition is often referred to as 'pseudoporphyria'. A screen for porphyrins should therefore be performed whenever blistering occurs in an apparently photosensitive distribution.

Epidermolysis bullosa acquisita

This is also extremely uncommon and closely resembles porphyria cutanea tarda clinically: blisters and fragility on trauma are seen on the backs of the hands, forearms, knees and shins. These heal, as in porphyria cutanea tarda, with scarring and milia formation. The diagnosis is largely one of exclusion, and porphyrins are negative. A number of patients with this disorder have had

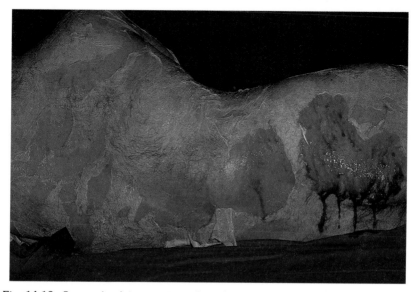

Fig. 14.12. Severe skin loss in toxic epidermal necrolysis.

associated diseases including various neoplasms, amyloidosis and inflammatory bowel disease.

Toxic epidermal necrolysis

The term 'toxic epidermal necrolysis' is applied to an acute onset of complete epidermal loss, usually over wide areas of the body surface, (Fig. 14.12) although localized forms have been described. Nikolsky's sign is positive. Primary toxic epidermal necrolysis may result from drug ingestion.

Such epidermal loss, whatever the cause, is a very serious matter. Patients become severely dehydrated and protein-depleted. They require intensive care and are best managed in a manner similar to burns patients.

Bullous erythema multiforme (Stevens–Johnson syndrome)

Erythema multiforme is a common reactional state which may follow a wide variety of triggers (see Chapter 15). In its most severe form, bullae may be the most prominent clinical feature. Occasionally this is so extensive that an appearance indistinguishable from toxic epidermal necrolysis can result.

Chapter 15
Miscellaneous Disorders

Miscellaneous:. . . of mixed composition or character; of various kinds; . . .
(The Concise Oxford Dictionary of Current English)

This chapter is a mixed bag: it covers a number of common and/or important skin disorders which need to be discussed but have not found a place elsewhere.

Urticaria and angioedema

The basic skin lesion of urticaria is a weal—a swelling of the skin which disappears leaving no visible sign. Most of us have personal experience of one common form of urticaria—after falling (or being pushed) into the nettles. Indeed 'nettle-rash' is a common lay term for urticaria.

The skin becomes irritable or stings and begins to swell. White lumps (weals) develop, which later become pink, often retaining a white rim around the edge. Lesions of urticaria can become very extensive and may appear in many sites at once. However, by definition the lesions also clear spontaneously within a few hours leaving no trace, even though other, new lesions may continue to develop. Typical lesions of urticaria are shown in Fig. 15.1.

The underlying pathology of a weal is oedema of the dermis. In some sites this oedema extends readily into the subcutaneous tissues—a situation known as 'angioedema'. Urticaria and angioedema often occur together. Sites of predilection for angioedema are around the eyes, the lips and in the oropharynx. These areas may swell alarmingly, occasionally resulting in complete closure of the eyes and compromising the airway. Oedema fluid accumulates in the skin or subcutis because blood vessels dilate and become leaky as a response to the release of histamine (and probably other mediators) following the degranulation of mast cells.

Clinical forms of urticaria and angioedema

Acute urticaria

Most attacks of urticaria last only a few hours or days. This may be due to contact with plants (e.g. nettles), animal fur (dogs, cats, horses) or foods (milk, egg white). Alternatively, widespread urticaria and/or angioedema may follow ingestion of certain foodstuffs and drugs. Common offenders include shellfish, strawberries (there is usually an outbreak at Wimbledon and Henley every summer), nuts, aspirin and penicillin. Atopic invidividuals are particularly prone to acute urticaria, which is generally triggered by IgE antibodies to the offending antigen. However, this is not always the case. Aspirin, for example, can initiate mast cell degranulation directly.

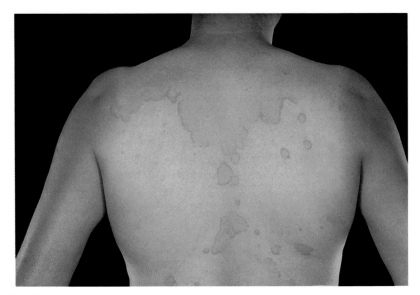

Fig. 15.1. Urticaria.

Chronic urticaria

Occasionally, attacks of urticaria may last for weeks or months. Contrary to popularly held opinion, it is usually not possible to demonstrate one single aetiological factor in this form of urticaria. Some authorities, especially in Scandinavia, maintain that chronic ingestion of food colourings and preservatives may be important, but in our experience (and that of others in the UK) this is only true of a minority of patients.

Physical urticaria

There are several physical insults which may trigger an urticarial response. Some are common, some extremely rare. The commonest is *dermographism,* in which weals appear after scratch-marks (Fig. 15.2). This may occur in isolation or in association with other forms of urticaria. *Cholinergic urticaria* is another common condition which largely affects young men. Small white weals with a red halo appear on the upper trunk after any stimulus which initiates sweating. Urticaria may also be triggered by *cold, water, sunlight,* and *heat.* There is also a rare form of urticaria in which weals develop some hours after *pressure.*

Hereditary angioedema

This is a very rare autosomal dominant condition in which the production of an enzyme (C1 esterase inhibitor) is either lacking or defective. Individuals are prone to sudden attacks of angioedema, which may extend throughout the gut, giving rise to abdominal pain. Gross swelling of the mouth and face may occur and be so severe as to be life-threatening.

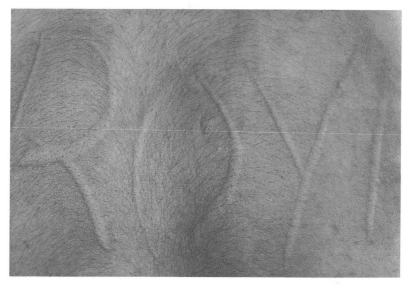

Fig. 15.2. Dermographism.

Urticaria pigmentosa

This is a rare disorder in which abnormal accumulations of mast cells give rise to multiple pigmented macules which urticate on being rubbed (see also Chapter 12).

Urticaria in systemic disease

Very occasionally an urticarial eruption may be part of a systemic disorder. For example, hepatitis B may present in this way, and the rash seen in the evenings in Still's disease is also urticarial in character (see Chapter 19).

Treatment of urticaria

If an underlying cause can be elicited from the history, this should obviously be avoided. It is sensible to ban aspirin for good in anyone prone to urticaria. If there is any suggestion of systemic disease this should be investigated.

Most types of urticaria respond in whole or in part to antihistamines, although some of the rarer forms are very resistant to therapy. The most useful agents are the H1 antagonists. There are now several non-sedative drugs in this class: terfenadine, astemizole, loratidine. There is no real need to treat urticaria with the older, sedative agents. Occasionally, it is worth adding an H2 antagonist (cimetidine, ranitidine) as well. For acute attacks, a few days' treatment is sufficient. For chronic urticaria the patient should be given a dose of antihistamine which suppresses the eruption completely and maintained on this for several months before gradually withdrawing the drug.

In an acute, severe attack with angioedema it may be necessary to use antihistamines parenterally. Very rarely, urticaria may accompany anaphylaxis and adrenaline may be required. Systemic steroids have a limited place, but may also assist in controlling severe urticaria.

Hereditary angioedema does not respond to antihistamines or steroids. The most appropriate management is with danazol which increases the levels of the missing enzyme.

Erythema multiforme

The classical finding in erythema multiforme is the 'iris' or 'target' lesion. This is a round or oval area of erythema, with a dusky, purplish centre (Fig. 15.3). Sometimes the central area of the lesion becomes paler and a blister forms. The lesions appear suddenly, enlarge over the course of a few days and may fade to leave pigmentary disturbance in their wake. The distribution is also characteristic; the extensor surfaces of arms and legs are prominently affected, but most important diagnostically is the involvement of palms and soles. Lesions normally continue to appear for about 3 weeks before the disorder spontaneously remits. Most patients have only one attack, but a few have repeated episodes especially in relation to herpes simplex (see below).

The underlying pathological process is a vasculitis and the more serious the vascular damage becomes, the more dramatic are the changes. With increasing degrees of severity, the epidermis becomes necrotic and fully separated from the underlying dermis. Bullae then become apparent clinically. It is not uncommon to see a few bullous lesions in relatively mild erythema multiforme, and it should always be considered in the differential diagnosis of blistering (see Chapter 14). However, when the inflammation and necrosis is very intense, bulla formation is the predominant clinical feature. When this occurs the disorder is often

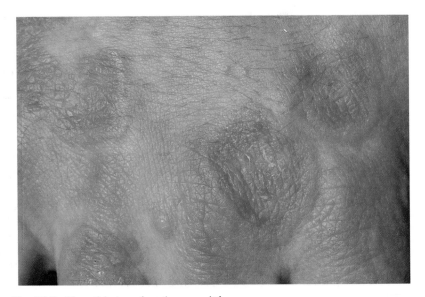

Fig. 15.3. 'Target' lesion of erythema multiforme.

known as 'Stevens–Johnson syndrome'. Mucous membrane changes may occur without skin lesions.

In Stevens–Johnson Syndrome there is a major systemic disturbance, with an acute onset of severe inflammation of eyes, mouth and genitalia (Fig. 15.4). In the mouth, blisters rapidly burst to leave severe erosions and patients are frequently unable to eat or drink. This may extend to the trachea and bronchial tree and patients occasionally die of severe bronchopneumonia. Renal failure may also occur. Sequelae such as ocular scarring and complete loss of nails may occur, although this is rare.

Erythema multiforme may occur out of the blue, but it may also be triggered by several drugs and disorders. The commonest of these is herpes simplex. As herpes may be recurrent, so may herpes-related erythema multiforme. Other potential triggers that are thought to be responsible occasionally include orf, hepatitis, mumps, a wide variety of drugs, radiotherapy, cancers and some connective tissue diseases.

Erythema multiforme is self-limiting and there is generally no need for treatment apart, perhaps, from antihistamines if there is significant pruritus. This is not true of the Stevens–Johnson syndrome. Close attention must be given to infection, fluid balance and nutrition, but the role of systemic steroids is controversial. Some maintain that the morbidity from steroids outweighs that of the underlying disease, which usually resolves without serious sequelae.

Exfoliative dermatitis (erythroderma)

The terms 'exfoliative dermatitis' or 'erythroderma' are used interchangeably to describe a specific clinical state in which the majority of the skin surface becomes red, inflamed and scaly (Fig. 15.5). There may be lymphadenopathy.

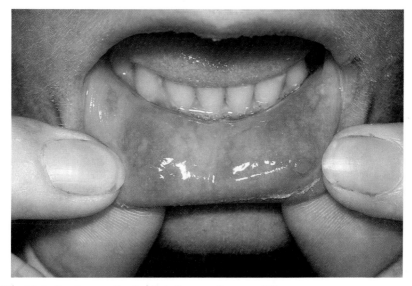

Fig. 15.4. Erosions on the lips in bullous erythema multiforme.

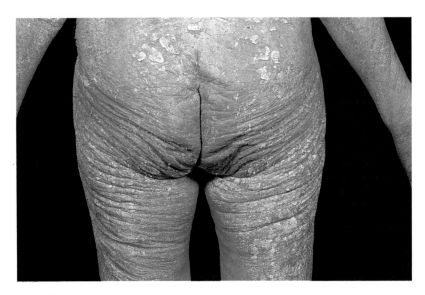

Fig. 15.5. Exfoliative dermatitis.

The effects of this state on the well-being of the body as a whole are considerable.

The most obvious result is that there is a loss of control of heat output. Patients with exfoliative dermatitis radiate heat into their surroundings. To compensate for this there is a general rise in metabolic rate, with mobilization of energy sources and increased muscle activity to conserve core temperature. Patients therefore have bouts of shivering. Cardiac output is markedly increased in order to supply blood to the inflamed skin. There is a gradual, inexorable loss of protein from the skin (and also the gut) and there is also a high water loss across the skin.

The body can only cope with all this for a limited period, especially in the elderly. Ultimately, there will be cardiac failure, renal failure or even sudden death due to central hypothermia. It is therefore important to diagnose and treat exfoliative dermatitis as soon as possible.

General management consists of ensuring that the patient is nursed in a warm room and is not allowed to get cold. It is obviously important to deal with any secondary medical problems such as dehydration, heart failure and infections. However, it is important to emphasize that exfoliative dermatitis is not a single pathological entity and that there are several important causes. Of these, four predominate: psoriasis; eczema/dermatitis; drug reactions; and lymphomas (especially cutaneous T cell lymphoma). It is vital in the correct management of exfoliative dermatitis that these are distinguished from each other, because the optimum treatment is different. It is important, for example, to stop any potential drug causes (see Chapter 21). Systemic steroids may be a useful short-term measure in eczema and drug reactions, but they are best avoided in psoriasis. Cutaneous involvement with lymphoma requires systemic investigation and appropriate treatment. If there is no preceding history of skin disease, therefore, a biopsy is essential.

Lichen planus

This is a relatively common skin disease. Classically, the disorder consists of an acute eruption of itchy papules. Individual lesions are flat-topped, shiny, tend to be polygonal in outline and are often a characteristic reddish purple colour, known as 'violaceous' after the violet family (Fig. 15.6). Lichen planus has a predilection for the wrists, ankles and the small of the back, but can occur anywhere. On the surface of the papules there is often a fine network of dots or lines which are called 'Wickham's striae'. Lichen planus also classically affects the mouth. Most commonly, there are lacy, reticulate streaks on the lining of the cheeks (Fig. 15.7), but similar changes may involve the gums and lips. There may be genital lesions too.

In the majority of patients, the eruption settles spontaneously over a period of a few months. Treatment with topical steroids is usually sufficient, although very extensive disease may require a short course of systemic steroids.

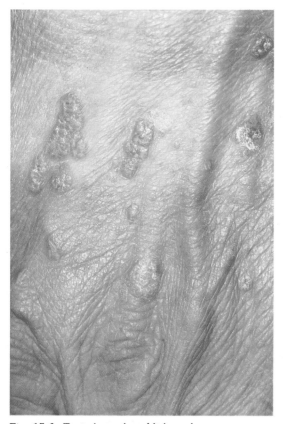

Fig. 15.6. Typical papules of lichen planus.

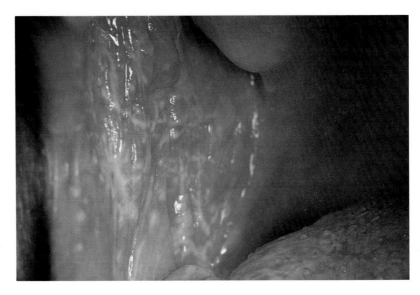

Fig. 15.7. Oral lesions in lichen planus.

There are also a number of rarer variants of lichen planus, in which the disease process adopts different clinical patterns. Of particular note are:

1 *Hypertrophic lichen planus* In this variant lichenified lumps appear on the legs.

2 *Atrophic lichen planus* This is largely seen in the mouth, where lesions may be very chronic and there is a slight risk of carcinoma.

3 *Follicular lichen planus* The disease affects hair, and may result in permanent scarring and hair loss.

4 *Lichen planus of the nails* Nail changes may be very slight or lead to complete destruction of the nail apparatus.

5 *Drug-induced lichen planus* This is covered in Chapter 21.

The pathological process in lichen planus appears to be a T cell mediated attack on the epidermis. Similar changes are seen in graft-versus-host reactions, and lichen planus can be triggered by drugs and sunlight. However, the cause of lichen planus in most instances remains a complete mystery.

Lichen nitidus

Considered by some to be a variant of lichen planus, this uncommon disorder produces an eruption of tiny, asymptomatic papules.

Lichen sclerosus et atrophicus

Lichen slcerosus et atrophicus (often shortened to lichen sclerosus) is a rare disorder of unknown aetiology with a marked predilection for the genitalia. It is, perhaps, important to note that there has been much confusion in the terminology of vulval disease, and that gynaecologists and dermatologists have traditionally used different labelling systems to describe vulval disease. However, it is now accepted by most authorities that lichen sclerosus has a special place in the nomenclature and is considered as a specific entity.

It is most common in women, in whom white patches appear on the vulva and may extend to involve the perianal skin. White, atrophic, scaly plaques may also develop on the skin. The surface of lesions may show purpura and occasionally blisters. Vulval lichen sclerosus also easily becomes eroded and haemorrhagic, frequently giving rise to symptoms of soreness and irritation. The disease in adults generally pursues a chronic, relapsing course. Topical steroids may provide symptomatic relief, but it is important to follow patients with lichen sclerosus carefully because there are two important complications: vaginal stenosis and neoplastic change, although the incidence of the latter is hard to estimate.

Lichen sclerosus may also occur in prepubertal girls, in whom it often presents with dysuria and pain on defaecation. It has also been confused with childhood sexual abuse. However, the lesions are clinically easy to diagnose (Fig. 15.8), and the parents and child reassured. The prognosis seems to be quite good in childhood disease, as a proportion clear at puberty.

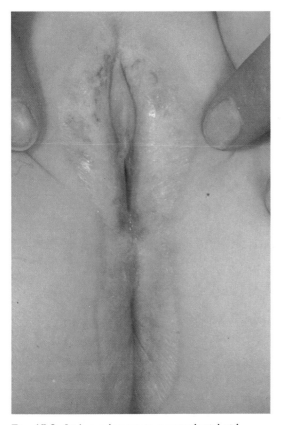

Fig. 15.8. Lichen sclerosus in a prepubertal girl.

Men and boys also develop lichen sclerosus. The changes are seen on the glans penis and prepuce, although extra-genital lesions may also occur. The ivory white plaques are sometimes called 'balanitis xerotica obliterans' and can give rise to phimosis and meatal stenosis. It is probable that a significant number of circumcisions for phimosis in boys are actually because of undiagnosed lichen sclerosus.

Pityriasis rosea

Pityriasis rosea is a relatively common self-limiting disorder predominantly affecting children and young adults. The cause is unknown, but a viral infection is suspected partly because it tends to occur in seasonal outbreaks and clusters and partly because it behaves like a rather lengthy viral exanthem. A full-blown and typical attack of pityriasis rosea is a very straightforward diagnosis because there are so many give-away signs.

There may or may not be a mild prodromal illness, but the first clue is the appearance of a large red, oval, scaly patch on the trunk or upper arm—the 'herald patch'. This is, of itself, easily confused with ringworm, eczema or psoriasis. However, a few days later, there is a sudden eruption of pink, oval patches on the trunk, upper arms and thighs. On the trunk these are arranged with their long axes in lines sweeping from the back to the front almost as if they were following spinal nerves (Fig. 15.9). This is said to give rise to an 'inverted

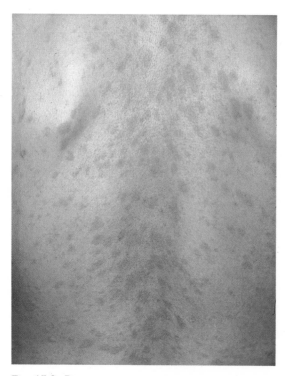

Fig. 15.9. Pityriasis rosea.

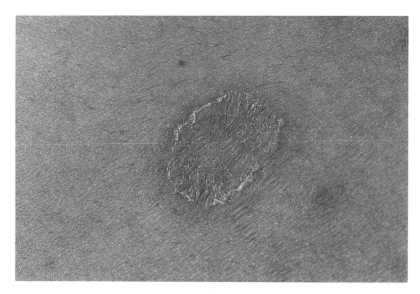

Fig. 15.10. Pityriasis rosea: the 'peripheral collarette' of scale.

Christmas tree' effect. Some find this confusing, partly because it depends on whether you are looking at the patient's back or front and partly because Christmas trees are often drawn wrongly! However, once understood, this sign should never be forgotten: no other disorder produces this appearance. The other classical feature to note is that the scale on the surface of each lesion exhibits a tendency to peel from the inside towards the edge, resulting in a so-called 'peripheral collarette' (Fig. 15.10).

Finally, if none of this has resulted in the diagnosis being made, it becomes clear that the rash was pityriasis rosea when it all disappears (as it always does) in about 6–8 weeks. Treatment is usually unecessary, but mild topical steroids may help to relieve irritation.

In saying that this is an easy disorder to diagnose, it has to be acknowledged that pityriasis rosea may present in an atypical manner: there may be no gap between the herald patch and the generalized rash; the eruption may extend down the arms and legs, and indeed occasionally spares the trunk altogether; lesions may be so numerous as to obliterate the neat distribution described above; the inflammation may be so intense as to cause blisters. However, once pityriasis rosea has been seen a few times, even these atypical forms will usually be recognized for what they are.

Pityriasis lichenoides

This is an uncommon condition in which small brownish red papules appear on the trunk and limbs. Classically the surface of each lesion is surmounted by a plate of scale which lifts off like mica. Some patients have more acutely inflamed lesions which heal to leave pock marks. Pityriasis lichenoides is commoner in children. Its cause is unknown but it is partially responsive to UV radiation.

Pityriasis rubra pilaris

Pityriasis rubra pilaris is a rare disease which occurs in localized or generalized forms. Lesions are reddish orange, sheeted and, as the name implies, involvement of hair follicles is a prominent feature. Localized lesions may give rise to confusion with psoriasis. Generalized pityriasis rubra pilaris is one of the rare causes of exfoliative dermatitis (see above).

Miliaria or 'prickly heat'

Miliaria rubra is the posh name for the little red bumps that some people get in hot conditions that induce sweating, especially where humidity is high. It is due to sweat duct obstruction. Patients complain of an acute 'prickling' in the affected areas. It should not be confused with polymorphic light eruption (see below) in which the lesions are induced by light not heat. The condition is also seen in infants, particularly affecting the napkin area.

Pregnancy rashes

Pregnancy may alter the course of a number of skin disorders, such as acne, eczema, psoriasis and vulval warts, and it may trigger erythema multiforme. There are also three important conditions that are specifically related to pregnancy itself: pruritus of pregnancy; polymorphic eruption of pregnancy; and herpes (pemphigoid) gestationis.

Pruritus is common in pregnancy. It is said that up to 20% of women suffer from it. Oestrogen-induced cholestasis may be responsible.

Polymorphic eruption of pregnancy is a characteristic, blotchy, urticarial and papular rash with intense irritation. Onset is usually in the third trimester, although it can be earlier. Some authorities recognize a separate early-onset

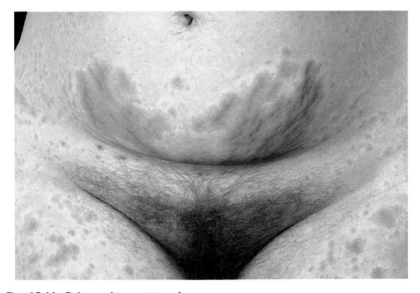

Fig. 15.11. Polymorphic eruption of pregnancy.

form: prurigo of pregnancy. The lesions of polymorphic eruption of pregnancy tend to begin on the abdomen (with a particular predilection for the striae—see Fig. 15.11). Later, the rash may become very widespread on the trunk and limbs. It fades shortly after delivery.

Herpes gestationis is very rare. Blisters develop on an urticated background. It seems to be a variant of bullous pemphigoid, triggered by pregnancy and there have been recent attempts to change its name to 'pemphigoid' gestationis.

Light-induced skin disease

But yet the light that led astray
Was light from Heaven
(Robert Burns, *The Vision*)

Light is often thought of as being good for you. Advertisements for sunbeds, solaria and foreign holidays all bear witness to this mid-twentieth century myth. However, there are a number of clinical situations in which UV radiation is important in initiating, wholly or in part, unwanted changes in the skin. Some changes are chronic, such as cancers, keratoses (see Chapter 9) and also the yellowing, coarsening and wrinkling known as 'photo-ageing', which is clearly related to long-term exposure to UV light. Many of today's tanned beauties are tomorrow's wrinkled prunes!

Some are more acute reactions, such as sunburn and reactions to a combination of plants or drugs and light. Some are due to metabolic disturbances, while in some the cause remains unknown. Ultraviolet may also cause a deterioration in certain pre-existing skin disorders (see below). This section deals with some of the more important of these reactions:

Sunburn
Polymorphic light eruption
Solar urticaria (see above)
Actinic prurigo
Juvenile spring eruption
Hyroa vacciniforme
Photosensitive eczema
Porphyrias
Pellagra
Xeroderma pigmentosum
Phytophotodermatitis
Drug reactions

Sunburn

Most of us are familiar with sunburn, even if we have only seen it in others. Excessive exposure to medium wavelength UV light (UVB) induces erythema and, if severe, blistering. The length of time required for this to happen depends largely on the skin type and pre-existing pigmentation (see Chapter 12) and on the intensity of the UV radiation. Skin Types I and II are very prone to sunburn, and UVB in sunlight around midday is at its most intense.

Treatment of established sunburn is difficult. Calamine lotion and topical steroids may help symptomatically, but the process tends to proceed inexorably, once established. Prevention is much better than cure. Sunscreens will generally prevent the development of sunburn, if used correctly. They should be applied to all exposed surfaces, and reapplied after swimming. Sunscreens come in a range of potencies, graded by 'Sun Protection Factor' (SPF) number. This number indicates the approximate multiple of time that the screen will provide: if your normal time to burn is 20 min, a screen with SPF 3 will prolong this to about an hour.

Polymorphic light eruption

This is a common disorder, which is frequently mis-diagnosed as 'prickly heat' (see above). Women are more affected than men, and typically trouble starts in adolescence or young adulthood. Patients notice that after being exposed to warm, sunny weather, they develop an eruption on light-exposed surfaces. Most commonly the areas affected are the face, arms, legs, and the 'V-neck' area of the trunk. The individual lesions are variable. In most instances they are papules, but larger plaques may develop and blisters are sometimes seen. For some this reaction only occurs in strong sunlight, for example when on a Mediterranean holiday, but others may develop a rash in weak British summer 'sunlight'.

The cause of polymorphic light eruption is completely unknown. Treament with preseason PUVA is helpful, and antimalarials may be of some benefit. Sunscreens and clothing will help prevent the eruption in some.

Actinic prurigo

Actinic prurigo is a rare disorder which starts in childhood. Eczematous areas develop on the face and backs of the hands every summer and disappear in the winter. The lesions may gradually begin to persist into the winter months, but they are usually much less severe. The cause is unknown and treatment is often a failure.

Juvenile spring eruption

Little boys occasionally develop blisters on the ears in the spring and this is given the grand title of juvenile spring eruption. It seems to stop happening after a while but it may be a 'forme-fruste' of polymorphic light eruption. It is important to distinguish this from *hydroa vacciniforme* a very rare disorder in which there is severe scarring. This tends to be a life-long problem.

Photosensitive eczema and chronic actinic dermatitis

Some individuals develop eczema of light-exposed surfaces which clears in the winter months. Some others have a pre-existing eczema which becomes much worse on exposure to light. In some this is due to a contact dermatitis to airborne chemicals, such as perfumes, or plant extracts. For example, one important cause of this pattern of skin change is chrysanthemums. A similar picture may occur with certain drugs. A careful history and investigation is therefore required in any patient who presents in this way.

However, in some the condition appears to be idiopathic and, as time goes by, the changes become more and more intense until the skin becomes permanently thickened and inflamed. This used to be called 'actinic reticuloid' because the histological changes resembled cutaneous lymphoma, but the term 'chronic actinic dermatitis' is now preferred. Treatment of this state is very difficult. Barrier sunscreens containing titanium may be helpful (if the patients will wear them), and azathioprine has been shown to be of benefit. However, this condition can completely ruin the quality of life because the sufferer may literally be unable to set foot outside without causing a deterioration in the state of his or her skin.

Porphyrias

This miscellaneous group of disorders are due to enzyme defects in the haem production pathways. Not all of them are associated with photosensitivity (e.g. acute intermittent porphyria, in which there are no skin signs at all). Porphyria cutanea tarda has already been mentioned in Chapter 14.The commonest cutaneous porphyria in Northern Europe is erythropoietic protoporphyria in which burning in the sun develops in early childhood. Light may continue to cause trouble through glass. This is an inherited condition in which the biochemical defect is at the very last stage of haem synthesis and blood protoporphyrin estimations are required for the diagnosis. Some patients find β-carotene helpful in preventing photosensitivity.

Variegate porphyria is seen amongst some Dutch and South African families, as well as very occasionally in other countries. It combines the general features of acute intermittent porphyria with the skin changes of porphyria cutanea tarda.

The other porphyrias are extremely rare. It is perhaps worth mentioning that erythropoietic porphyria (Gunther's disease) may have been the origin of the legend of the werewolf. This is because sufferers become disfigured and hairy, are anaemic (and therefore crave blood?) and because they can only go out at night (and before the days of street lights they could only see where they were going when the moon was full!).

Pellagra

Pellagra is an important cause of a photosensitive rash in the malnourished. There is a classical triad: Diarrhoea, Dermatitis and Dementia. In Western societies this is only seen in alcoholics and recluses.

Xeroderma pigmentosum

This rare disorder often presents with photosensitivity in early childhood (see also Chapter 11).

Phytophotodermatitis

Every summer, we see patients who have developed a rash following contact with plants on sunny days. This produces typical linear, streaky dermatitis

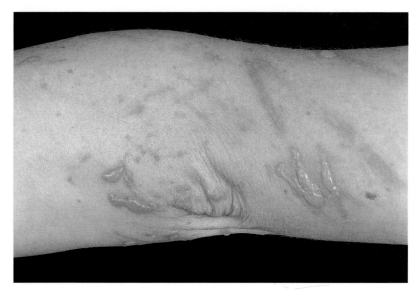

Fig. 15.12. A phytophotodermatitis.

(Fig. 15.12). Residual pigmentary disturbances are common. One important cause is giant hogweed, but there are several other offenders.

Light-induced drug reactions

Several groups of drugs are associated with photo-allergic and phototoxic reactions (see Chapter 21).

Disorders exacerbated by light

There are also a number of disorders which may show a deterioration or provocation by exposure to light:

    Lupus erythematosus
    Rosacea
    Psoriasis
    Darier's disease
    Herpes simplex

The mechanisms for this are unclear.

Chapter 16
Vascular Disorders

Leg ulcers

By far the commonest type of leg ulcer is the venous ulcer. Other causes of leg ulceration include ischaemia, vasculitis, skin neoplasia, and certain haematological disorders.

Venous hypertension and venous leg ulcers
(varicose ulcers; stasis ulcers; gravitational ulcers)

Venous return from the legs is dependent on the calf muscle pump pushing blood from the deep veins upwards towards the heart. Valves in the deep veins prevent reflux of blood when the muscle pump is relaxed. Venous hypertension is the result of incompetent valves and as a consequence of this an ineffective calf muscle pump. Congenital abnormalities of the venous system, and valve damage during recanalization following episodes of deep vein thrombosis, may contribute to incompetence of the valves. Genetic factors are probably important, as certain racial groups have a low incidence of venous hypertension and its accompanying manifestations.

The high pressure in the deep veins of the legs is transmitted via incompetent perforating veins to the superficial venous system, resulting in dilated, tortuous 'varicose' veins. Skin capillaries also become dilated and tortuous, and 'leaky'. Plasma passes through the vascular endothelium into the pericapillary tissues, where fibrinogen is converted to fibrin, which forms cuffs around the blood vessels. It is also possible that leukocyte stasis in capillaries leads to release of enzymes which damage vascular endothelium, increasing its permeability, and that this mechanism contributes to leakage of vessel contents into surrounding tissues. These changes result in tissue hypoxia, and this relatively devitalized tissue is susceptible to ulceration, either spontaneously or following minor trauma.

The problems caused by venous hypertension usually present in middle or old age, and women, particularly the obese, are predominantly affected. The clinical features include:

1 *Oedema.*

2 *Lipodermatosclerosis* This term is applied to areas of induration, caused by fibrosis, on the lower parts of the legs, above the ankles (Fig. 16.1). The affected areas are often erythematous initially, but eventually they become purple-brown in colour. When lipodermatosclerosis is circumferential the tissues above the ankle are constricted, giving the leg the classical inverted champagne bottle appearance.

3 *Hyperpigmentation* Haemosiderin, derived from red cells extravasated from dilated, leaky capillaries, produces areas of brown discolouration of the skin.

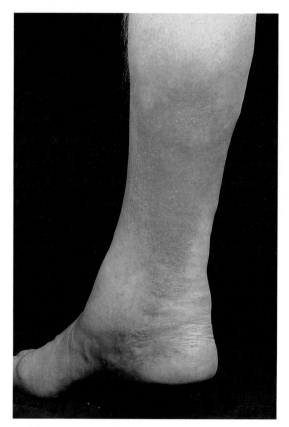

Fig. 16.1. Lipodermatosclerosis.

4 *Eczema* Areas of 'varicose' eczema on the legs are common in patients suffering from venous hypertension.

5 *Atrophie blanche* This term is applied to areas of scar tissue within which are prominent dilated capillaries. The appearance is of scattered pink dots on a white background (Fig. 16.2). Areas of atrophie blanche are very prone to ulcerate, and usually the ulcers, although relatively small, are extremely painful, in contrast to the majority of large venous leg ulcers.

6 *Ulcers* The commonest site for a venous ulcer is the medial aspect of the leg, just above the medial malleolus (Fig. 16.3), but the lateral malleolar area may also be affected. Venous ulcers are often surrounded by areas of lipodermatosclerosis and varicose eczema.

Rarely, a squamous cell epithelioma may develop in a long-standing venous ulcer.

Treatment

Lipodermatosclerosis, if treated early, may respond to the fibrinolysis-enhancing agent stanozolol (Stromba). Varicose eczema may be treated with mild potency topical steroids or medicated bandages such as Viscopaste or Ichthopaste.

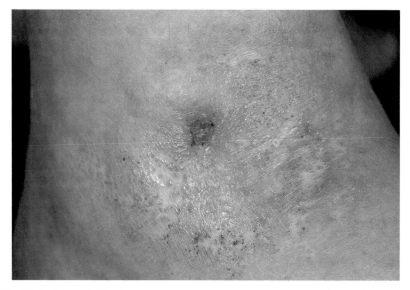

Fig. 16.2. Atrophie blanche.

Weight reduction in the obese will also help, in theory, but in practice this is usually extremely difficult to achieve or to maintain. Vein surgery is only of value in a small number of cases.

When venous ulcers are present, the single most important aspect of management is to keep oedema to a minimum by good compression bandaging or graduated compression stockings. Diuretic therapy may also help. Far too much attention is usually paid to topical therapy of the ulcer, and not enough

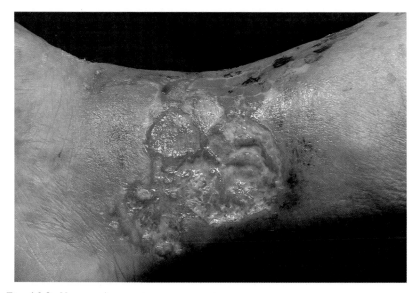

Fig. 16.3. Venous ulcer.

to increasing the efficiency of the calf muscle pump and eliminating oedema. This aspect of treatment is just as vital after the ulcers have healed, but is often neglected, with the result that ulcers rapidly recur. The list of topical agents available for the treatment of leg ulcers is long and varied. Some are designed to kill bacteria, some to absorb exudate, some to neutralize odour, some to de-slough, and some to stimulate granulation tissue production. None will provide a great deal of benefit unless some attempt is made to eliminate oedema and restore the function of the muscle pump.

A typical venous ulcer requires cleaning every few days with saline, followed by the application of a topical antibacterial such as povidone iodine (Betadine) or silver sulphadiazine (Flamazine). Adherent slough may be physically removed with tweezers and scissors, or by a de-sloughing agent such as streptokinase/streptodornase (Varidase). If, after regular cleaning, there is little sign of granulation tissue formation, a hydrocolloid dressing such as Granuflex may help to stimulate granulation. When an ulcer is clean and granulating, healing may be accelerated by grafting. A simple type of skin grafting procedure is pinch-grafting, in which small pieces of skin, usually taken from the thigh, are scattered over the surface of the ulcer (Fig. 16.4). The end result is a rather mammillated surface, but the cosmetic appearance is not important. Larger ulcers will require more extensive partial-thickness grafting.

Topical antibiotic preparations containing neomycin should not be used on venous ulcers because of the tendency of neomycin to cause allergic contact dermatitis.

There is no ideal preparation to heal venous ulcers. The best results are always obtained by those willing to lavish abundant tender loving care on the sufferers.

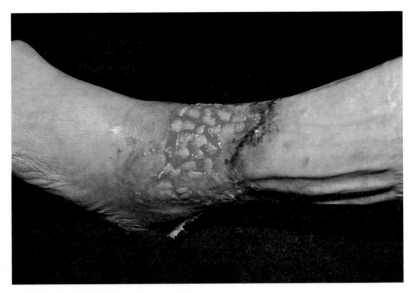

Fig. 16.4. Pinch grafts on a venous ulcer.

Ischaemic ulcers

Ischaemic ulceration is usually a manifestation of atherosclerotic peripheral vascular disease. Typically, ischaemic ulcers occur on the dorsum or the sides of the foot, between the toes, or on the heel. Pedal pulses are absent. Ischaemic ulcers are usually painful.

Treatment

The advice of a vascular surgeon should be sought in the management of ischaemic ulceration. Arterial surgery may help a few cases, and occasionally sympathectomy may increase skin blood flow and encourage healing. In many cases, however, ischaemic ulceration is progressive, and necessitates amputation.

Vasculitis

Necrotizing vasculitis associated with a number of disorders, including rheumatoid arthritis and systemic lupus erythematosus (SLE) may produce ulceration on the legs.

Neoplastic ulcers

Basal cell carcinomas and squamous cell carinomas arising on the legs may resemble, and be mistaken for, venous leg ulcers. However, they usually occur above the ankle region, and neoplasia should be considered as a possibility in ulcers developing higher up the leg. If there is any doubt, a biopsy should be performed.

Haematological disorders and leg ulcers

Uncommon causes of leg ulcers include hereditary spherocytosis, sickle cell anaemia and thalassaemia. The mechanism of ulceration in these conditions is related to tissue hypoxia due to blockage of skin capillaries by abnormally-shaped red cells.

Vasculitis

Vascular inflammation may be classified according to the type of immunological reaction responsible for its production, the clinical appearance of the lesions, or the pathological changes visible on histology. As a result, it is easy to become completely confused by terminology, and to wish that you were reading about something else.

Immunologically, Type III (immune complex) and Type IV (cell-mediated, delayed hypersensitivity) reactions are responsible for the majority of vasculitic disease. Clinically, vasculitis may present as urticaria, livedo reticularis, purpuric papules, nodules, haemorrhagic bullae or ulcers. Histologically, the changes are related to the immunological mechanisms responsible for the reaction, and can be classified as leukocytoclastic (immune-complex mediated; polymorphs predominate in the infiltrate), lymphocytic (delayed hypersensitivity; lymphocytes predominate), and granulomatous (immune-complex mediated; perivascular granuloma formation).

Clinical presentations of vasculitis

'Allergic' vasculitis (necrotizing vasculitis: leukocytoclastic vasculitis)

Typically, an affected individual presents with multiple palpable, purpuric lesions on the legs, predominantly below the knees (Fig. 16.5). Some lesions may develop into haemorrhagic vesicles or bullae. Histologically there is fibrinoid necrosis of small blood vessels, and a perivascular infiltrate composed predominantly of neutrophil polymorphs. The perivascular tissues also contain extravasated red cells, and fragments of polymorph nuclei ('nuclear dust'). These changes are initiated by deposition of immune complexes in small vessels, complement activation, and production of polymorph chemotactic factors. Polymorphs attracted to the area release lysosomal enzymes which damage the vessel wall. Drugs, bacterial and viral infections may act as the antigenic triggers for this type of reaction, but often the initiating factor is not discovered. This type of vasculitis may also be associated with rheumatoid arthritis, SLE and Sjögren's syndrome.

In many cases there is no evidence of systemic vascular involvement, but the joints, kidneys and gastrointestinal tract may be affected.

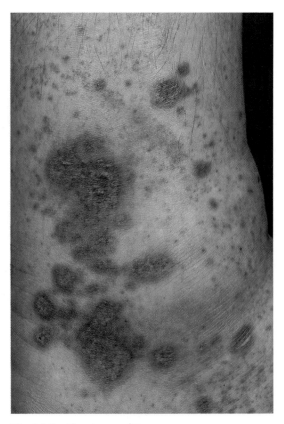

Fig. 16.5. Allergic vasculitis.

Henoch–Schönlein purpura (anaphylactoid purpura) is the name which has been given to a systemic allergic vasculitis occurring predominantly in children. Palpable purpuric lesions on the buttocks and legs are associated with arthralgia, gastrointestinal symptoms, vomiting and bloody diarrhoea, and proliferative glomerulonephritis. In many cases the precipitating factor appears to be a streptococcal sore throat.

Treatment A period of bed rest may result in complete resolution of the skin lesions. In some cases, however, recurrent crops of lesions occur, and these may respond to therapy with dapsone. Dapsone does not affect immune complex formation, it simply blocks the pathomechanics of the production of skin lesions. In more severe cases, particularly those with systemic involvement, systemic steroid therapy may be necessary.

Polyarteritis nodosa

Polyarteritis nodosa (also known as periarteritis nodosa) is an uncommon type of necrotizing vasculitis which affects medium-sized arteries throughout the body. Its aetiology is unknown in the majority of cases, but it may be provoked by hepatitis B infection. Middle-aged men are affected predominantly. Affected blood vessels show fibrinoid necrosis, a perivascular neutrophil infiltrate and nuclear dust. Vessel damage results in aneurysm formation. Manifestations include pyrexia, weight loss, arthralgia and myalgia. Most affected individuals have a mild anaemia, leukocytosis, eosinophilia, and a high erythrocyte sedimentation rate (ESR) or raised plasma viscosity. In some, circulating immune complexes can be demonstrated. Skin lesions include nodules (produced by vasculitis affecting small and medium-sized arteries), livedo reticularis, and ulcers. Renal involvement leads to hypertension, proteinuria, haematuria and renal failure. Nervous system involvement is common, and is frequently manifest as peripheral neuropathy or mononeuritis multiplex. Dysrhythmias and myocardial ischaemia denote cardiac involvement, and gut involvement may be manifest as gastrointestinal haemorrhage.

There is a type of polyarteritis nodosa which affects the skin alone. Cutaneous nodules and livedo reticularis occur on the legs, usually below the knees, and there is no evidence of systemic involvement.

Treatment Polyarteritis nodosa is treated with systemic steroids and immunosuppressive drugs. High doses of systemic steroids may be required to control the condition. The prognosis is variable, and there is a significant mortality in spite of treatment.

Cutaneous polyarteritis nodosa follows a benign course, and is usually responsive to small doses of systemic steroids.

Erythema nodosum

This condition usually affects children and young adults, and is characterized by the development of multiple tender, erythematous nodules, usually on the shins (Fig. 16.6), but occasionally also on the forearms. As each nodule regresses it

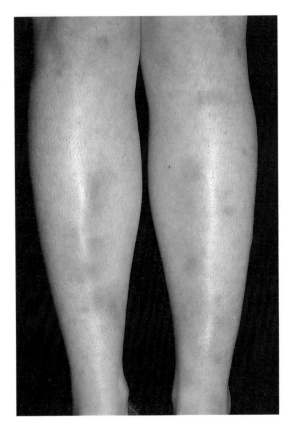

Fig. 16.6. Erythema nodosum.

changes colour from red to purple to yellow-green—like a fading bruise. Pathologically, erythema nodosum is a nodular panniculitis associated with a lymphocytic vasculitis.

Erythema nodosum may be provoked by a number of stimuli, including:
1 Streptococcal infection.
2 Drugs: particularly sulphonamides.
3 Sarcoidosis.
4 Primary tuberculosis.
5 Inflammatory bowel disease.
In some cases no precipitating factor is discovered.

Investigation of a patient suffering from erythema nodosum should include a throat swab, ASO titre, chest X-ray, Mantoux test, and Kveim test if the Mantoux is negative.

Treatment In many cases of erythema nodosum bed rest and simple analgesia is all that is required. The lesions will gradually resolve over a period of a few days.

Temporal arteritis (giant cell arteritis)

This is a disease of the elderly, of unknown aetiology, in which a focal granulomatous vasculitis affects medium-sized and large arteries throughout the body. It is the cranial arteries, however, which are responsible for most of the symptomatology. Severe, often bilateral, headache is accompanied by tenderness of the skin over the temporal and parietal regions of the scalp, and the skin in these areas may become necrotic and ulcerate. The superficial temporal arteries are tender and swollen. Involvement of vessels supplying the jaw and the tongue may result in jaw and lingual claudication. Involvement of the retinal arteries may be manifest as transient visual impairment, ischaemic optic neuritis, or sudden blindness due to arterial occlusion. The ESR is markedly elevated, and temporal artery biopsy will show the typical changes.

Treatment If temporal arteritis is suspected, the patient should be treated immediately with a high dose of systemic steroids. Delay could mean permanent loss of vision.

Wegener's granulomatosis

This is a rare form of necrotizing granulomatous vasculitis affecting principally the small arteries of the respiratory tract, and associated with glomerulonephritis. The disease usually presents with upper respiratory tract problems, in the form of chronic sinusitis, rhinorrhoea and epistaxis. The lungs are frequently involved, and chest X-ray usually reveals multiple nodular opacities. Glomerulonephritis occurs in the majority of patients. Skin lesions take the form of a nodular vasculitis, sometimes with ulceration.

Treatment Untreated, the prognosis is very poor. Treatment with systemic steroids and cyclophosphamide dramatically improves the prognosis.

Pyoderma gangrenosum
(See Chapter 19.)

Behçet's syndrome

In 1937 Behçet described a clinical triad of recurrent oral and genital ulceration and uveitis. Subsequently, a number of other manifestations, including non-erosive arthritis, skin lesions (erythema nodosum; pustular lesions), thrombophlebitis, neurological disease (aseptic meningitis; cranial nerve palsies; cerebellar disease), and colitis have been described. The disease usually affects young adults, and appears to be more prevalent in eastern Mediterranean countries and Japan. The basic pathological process in Behçet's syndrome is a vasculitis principally involving veins and venules.

Treatment The mainstay of treatment for Behçet's syndrome is systemic steroids. Other drugs which may be of benefit in some cases include colchicine, azathioprine and chlorambucil.

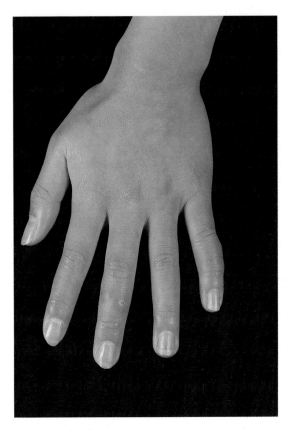

Fig. 16.7. Chilblains.

Perniosis (chilblains)

Chilblains are painful, inflammatory lesions provoked by exposure to cold (Fig. 16.7). The commonest sites for chilblains are the fingers and toes, but they may also occur on fatty prominences such as the fat pads on the medial aspects of the knees, and on the thighs. A characteristic type of perniosis occurs during winter months on the lateral aspect of the thighs in those fond of equestrian pursuits, particularly if the thighs happen to be rather ample, and covered only by thin jodhpurs (equestrian cold panniculitis).

Treatment for chilblains is not very satisfactory, the best management being prophylaxis, by wearing warm gloves and thick socks, and, in the case of the equestrian, thermal underwear.

Chapter 17
Connective Tissue Disorders

Lupus erythematosus

Lupus erythematosus is an autoimmune disorder which occurs in two main forms: systemic lupus erythematosus (SLE) which affects both the skin and internal organs; and discoid lupus erythematosus (DLE) in which the skin alone is affected. A small proportion of patients suffering from DLE may subsequently develop SLE.

Systemic lupus erythematosus (SLE)

This is a multisystem disorder which may affect the skin, joints, heart and pericardium, lungs, kidneys, brain and haemopoietic system. Typically, the disease affects women, particularly of childbearing age, and progresses in a series of exacerbations and remissions. Its aetiology is unknown.

Mucocutaneous lesions encountered in SLE include oropharnygeal ulceration, diffuse alopecia, Raynaud's phenomenon, and photosensitivity. Often there is characteristic facial erythema in a 'butterfly' distribution (Fig. 17.1). The wings of the 'butterfly' are represented by erythema on the cheeks, and they are linked by a band of erythema extending across the nasal bridge. Other diseases may produce butterfly erythema on the face, and by far the commonest cause of this pattern of facial erythema is rosacea. Cutaneous vasculitis occurs in SLE and may be manifest as microinfarcts on the digits, multiple vasculitic lesions on the legs, or an urticaria-like eruption known as urticarial vasculitis.

Systemic manifestations include:

1 Polyserositis:
 (a) Arthralgia and arthritis (usually non-erosive).
 (b) Pericarditis.
 (c) Pleurisy with effusions.
2 Glomerulonephritis.
3 Central nervous system involvement—psychosis and convulsions.
4 Haemopoietic abnormalities:
 (a) Normochromic, normocytic anaemia.
 (b) Coombs' positive haemolytic anaemia.
 (c) Leukopenia.
 (d) Thrombocytopenia (associated with antiplatelet antibodies).
5 Pyrexia, weight loss and general malaise.

Investigations

Antinuclear antibodies (ANA), also known as antinuclear factor (ANF), and DNA antibodies are found in the majority of patients suffering from SLE. Antibodies to double-stranded DNA are characteristic of lupus. A number of

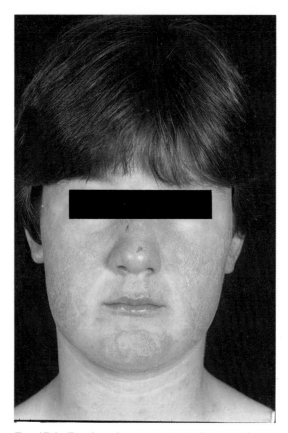

Fig. 17.1. Facial erythema in systemic lupus erythematosus.

other autoantibodies may occur in patients with SLE including: anti-Ro, anti-La, antibodies to extractable nuclear antigen, lymphocytotoxic antibodies, and the lupus anticoagulant. A positive rheumatoid factor and biological false positive serological tests for syphilis may be found in some patients with SLE.

Direct immunofluorescence performed on skin biopsies from clinically involved areas of skin shows linear deposition of IgG or IgM, and C3 at the dermoepidermal junction. Immunoglobulin and complement deposition may also be demonstrable in biopsies taken from normal skin in light-exposed areas.

Treatment

Mild SLE without significant renal or CNS involvement may be managed with non-steroidal anti-inflammatory drugs or antimalarial therapy. Severe SLE will require treatment with systemic steroids and immunosuppressive agents such as azathioprine. Plasmapheresis may also produce temporary benefit in severe cases. Light-exposed areas of skin should be protected by the use of sunscreens with a high sun protection factor (SPF).

Prognosis

Severe renal and CNS involvement are poor prognostic factors, but for the majority of cases of SLE the prognosis is good with present treatment regimes.

Drug-induced SLE

Drug-induced SLE is rare. The drugs most frequently implicated in provocation of SLE include: hydrallazine, procainamide, anticonvulsants (phenytoin, primidone), isoniazid and chlorpromazine.

Discoid lupus erythematosus

Classically, discoid lupus erythematosus (DLE) affects the light-exposed areas—principally the face and neck, but the dorsa of the hands and the arms may also be affected. Lesions may be precipitated or exacerbated by sunlight. Individual lesions consist of scaling, erythematous plaques, with prominent follicular plugging. If the scale is lifted off, the follicular plugs may be seen on its undersurface—the so-called 'carpet-tack' appearance. There may be only a few lesions, but in severe cases there is extensive, cosmetically disfiguring involvement of the facial skin. Lesions heal with scarring, and the typical picture in an established case of DLE is of an active, erythematous scaly margin enclosing a central area of scarred, hypopigmented, atrophic skin (Fig. 17.2). The scalp may be involved, producing areas of scarring alopecia, in which follicles are permanently destroyed. Occasionally the buccal or nasal mucosae are affected.

Investigations

The clinical appearance is typical in the majority of cases, but the diagnosis can be confirmed by skin biopsy. Histology shows a periadnexal lymphocytic infiltrate, liquefaction degeneration of the basal layer of the epidermis, follicular plugging and hyperkeratosis. Direct immunofluorescence of lesional skin reveals the same pattern of immunoglobulin deposition seen in SLE, i.e. linear deposition of IgG or IgM at the dermoepidermal junction, producing the so-called lupus band. The ANF may be positive, but DNA antibodies are not present in significant amounts.

Treatment

Potent fluorinated topical steroids are frequently helpful in the management of DLE. In cases not responding to topical steroids intralesional injection of triamcinolone, or oral therapy with the antimalarial hydroxychloroquine may be of benefit. Exposure to strong sunlight should be avoided, and light-exposed areas protected by use of a sunscreen with a high SPF. In cases where there is extensive involvement of facial skin, the use of cosmetic camouflage creams can produce a considerable improvement in the appearance of the skin.

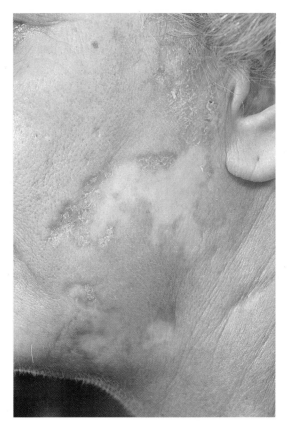

Fig. 17.2. Discoid lupus erythematosus.

Dermatomyositis

Heliotrope
A flower resembling the pale violet,
Which, with the Sun, though rooted-fast, doth move
And, being changed, yet changeth not her love.

(Ovid)

Dermatomyositis is an autoimmune inflammatory disease of skin and muscle. It is closely related to polymyositis which has all the muscle features of dermatomyositis, but no skin involvement. Dermatomyositis may occur in childhood or in adult life, and there are certain differences in the manifestations of the disease in these two age groups. The occurrence of vasculitis and the late development of calcinosis are features of the childhood disease which are not seen in adults, and in some adults dermatomyositis is associated with systemic malignancy, whereas there is no such association in the childhood disease.

Clinical features

Skin The characteristic skin changes seen in dermatomyositis are as follows:

1 Erythema of the face and V-area of the neck (Fig. 17.3). The facial skin may have a violaceous hue, particularly in childhood dermatomyositis, said to resemble the colour of the Heliotrope flower, and referred to as 'heliotrope erythema' (Greek scholars will realize that Heliotrope means 'turning towards the sun').

2 Periorbital oedema.

3 Erythema on the dorsa of the hands, and linear erythema on the dorsa of the fingers (Fig. 17.4). There may be erythematous papules (Gottron's papules) over the knuckles.

4 Prominent, ragged cuticles and dilated capillaries in the proximal nail folds.

5 Erythema over knees and elbows.

6 In the childhood disease, cutaneous vasculitis leads to ulceration of the skin, particularly in the axillae and groins.

Muscles Muscle involvement is variable. In some cases there is little evidence of any muscle disease, whereas in others there is profound muscle weakness. Typically, there is proximal, symmetrical weakness and wasting of the limb girdle muscles. Pharyngeal and oesophageal muscles may also be involved, leading to dysphagia.

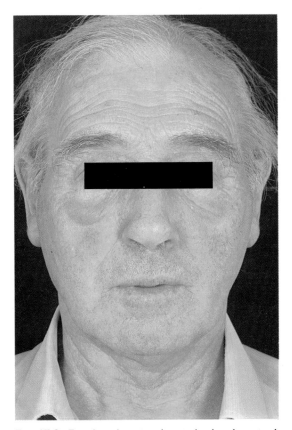

Fig. 17.3. Facial erythema and periorbital oedema in dermatomyositis.

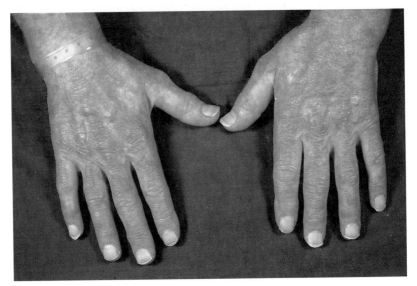

Fig. 17.4. Linear erythema on the dorsa of the hands in dermatomyositis.

Other features in some patients suffering from dermatomyositis include pulmonary fibrosis, and arthralgia and/or arthritis.

There have been a number of studies of the association between adult dermatomyositis and systemic malignancy, and these have produced some controversy about the prevalence of this association. There is no doubt that some adult patients suffering from dermatomyositis have an underlying systemic malignancy, but there is no general agreement as to how frequently this association occurs. There is also disagreement over the necessity for an extensive search for an occult neoplasm in a patient with dermatomysitis, but several studies have suggested that extensive screening for occult neoplasia is of little value. However, should a patient with dermatomyositis develop pulmonary or abdominal symptomatology this should be thoroughly investigated.

Investigations

Electromyography and biopsy of affected muscles, measurement of serum enzymes (creatine kinase; aldolase) derived from muscle, and a 24-h urine creatine level, will help to confirm the diagnosis.

Treatment

In those cases of dermatomyositis associated with an underlying malignancy there is usually marked improvement when the neoplasm is excised. A relapse of the dermatomyositis signals a recurrence or the development of metastatic malignancy, and in these cases the prognosis is usually poor.

The mainstay of drug therapy for dermatomyositis is oral corticosteroids. In patients whose response to steroids is poor, immunosuppressives such as azathioprine, methotrexate, cyclophosphamide or chlorambucil may be of benefit. Where there is severe muscle involvement regular physiotherapy is an important adjunct to drug therapy, in order to minimize contractures resulting from progressive muscle fibrosis.

Scleroderma

The term scleroderma means thickening of the skin, and is applied to a group of diseases in which there is sclerosis of the skin with destruction of hair follicles and sweat glands. Scleroderma may be an isolated cutaneous phenomenon, when it is called 'morphoea', or a cutaneous component of a multisystem disorder.

Classification of scleroderma

1 *Morphoea* Sclerosis of the skin without systemic involvement.

2 *Systemic sclerosis* Cutaneous sclerosis in association with a vasculopathy of small arteries producing multi-organ systemic disease.

3 *Chemically-induced scleroderma* Sclerosis of the skin as a manifestation of the toxic effects of certain chemicals.

4 *Pseudoscleroderma* Sclerosis of the skin associated with a number of diseases other than morphoea or systemic sclerosis.

Morphoea

This is a disorder of unknown aetiology in which there is sclerosis of the skin. Morphoea may be subdivided clinically into the following types:

1 Circumscribed.

2 Linear.

3 Frontoparietal (en coup de sabre).

4 Generalized.

1 *Circumscribed* This is the commonest clinical presentation of morphoea. Indurated plaques, which may be solitary or multiple, develop spontaneously, predominantly on the trunk. Initially the affected areas of skin have a violaceous hue, but gradually they become thickened and ivory in colour (Fig. 17.5). The surface is smooth and shiny, and because the pathological process destroys hair follicles and sweat glands the plaques are devoid of hair and do not sweat. Eventually, usually after many months, the sclerosis resolves, leaving atrophic, hyperpigmented areas.

2 *Linear* Linear morphoea usually affects one limb as an area of linear sclerosis, often extending the full length of the limb. Linear morphoea occurring in childhood can signficantly impair the growth of a limb, and also produce severe flexion deformities of large joints and digits.

3 *Frontoparietal (en coup de sabre)* Resembling a sabre cut across the scalp and forehead, this type of morphoea is a considerable cosmetic problem. A linear, depressed, sclerotic area extends from the face into the scalp, and is associated with loss of hair over the affected area.

4 *Generalized* There is extensive sclerosis of the skin of the trunk and limbs. In the most severe cases involvement extends from the scalp to the toes. Flexion

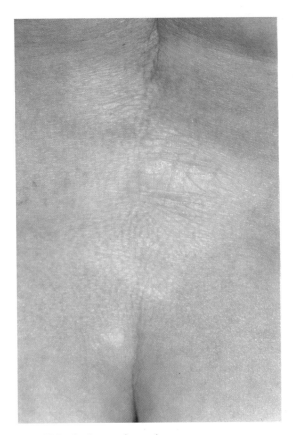

Fig. 17.5. A plaque of morphoea.

contractures restrict limb movement, and if the chest is severely affected breathing may be impaired. Interestingly, the areolae and nipples are not affected by the sclerotic process.

Treatment of morphoea

There is no really effective treatment for morphoea. There is evidence that some cases of linear morphoea in childhood benefit from treatment with penicillamine, but in the majority of cases of morphoea drug therapy is ineffective. Physiotherapy is essential in the management of linear morphoea on the limbs, and orthopaedic surgery may be necessary to correct joint contractures. Plastic surgery may be of help in cases of frontoparietal morphoea.

The natural history of morphoea is a process of gradual spontaneous resolution.

Systemic sclerosis

This is a condition of unknown aetiology in which sclerotic changes in the skin occur as one component of a multisystem disorder associated with a vasculopathy of small arteries. The skin changes affect predominantly the face and hands, and include:

Face
1 The facial skin is sclerotic and bound to underlying structures, producing a tight, shiny appearance, with loss of facial wrinkles, a beaked nose, and constriction of the mouth opening (Fig. 17.6).
2 Peri-oral furrowing ('purse-string mouth').
3 Facial telangiectasia.
4 Loss of lip vermillion.

Hands
1 Raynaud's phenomenon.
2 Tight sclerotic skin producing progressive contractures of the digits (sclerodactyly).
3 Finger pulp infarcts producing small, painful ulcers (Fig. 17.7). These infarctive changes lead to progressive pulp atrophy and resorption of the underlying terminal phalanges.
4 Calcinosis.

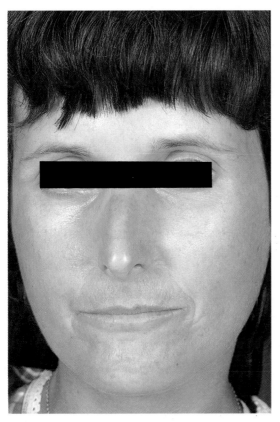

Fig. 17.6. Facial appearance in systemic sclerosis.

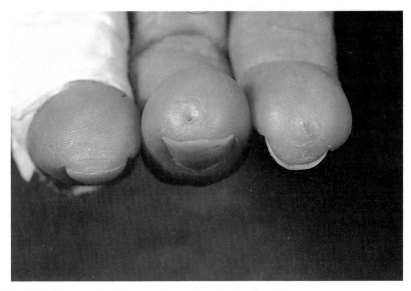

Fig. 17.7. Finger pulp ulcers and scars in systemic sclerosis.

Persistant leg ulcers, predominantly affecting the ankles, are not uncommon in systemic sclerosis.

Systemic involvement

Gastrointestinal There is atrophy and fibrosis of the circular smooth muscle of the oesophagus, resulting in impaired peristalsis. The gastro-oesophageal sphincter mechanism is also impaired, leading to gastro-oesophageal reflux, oesophagitis, and eventually to stricture formation. Symptoms of oesophageal reflux are common. Dysphagia usually indicates the development of oesophageal stricture. Barium swallow in the Trendelenberg position (head down) and oesophageal manometry will demonstrate oesophageal dysfunction.

Atrophy and fibrosis of the smooth muscle of the small bowel leads to impaired peristalsis, and the resulting stagnation of small bowel contents predisposes to bacterial overgrowth. Gut bacteria deconjugate bile salts, which are essential for micelle formation, and this leads to fat malabsorption and steatorrhoea. Occasionally, patients with small bowel involvement present with a picture simulating acute intestinal obstruction.

The typical change seen in the large bowel is the presence of multiple wide-mouthed sacculations (pseudodiverticula).

Symptomatically patients with gut involvement may complain of either constipation or diarrhoea.

Pulmonary Pulmonary disease in systemic sclerosis usually has an insidious onset with gradually increasing shortness of breath, and takes the form of pulmonary fibrosis and pulmonary hypertension. The latter is due to disease of small pulmonary arteries, and eventually leads to cor pulmonale.

Renal Pathological changes resembling those seen in severe hypertension i.e. fibrinoid changes in arteries and arterioles, are associated with proteinuria and hypertension. In the majority of cases of systemic sclerosis renal involvement is mild, but in a few it is rapidly progressive and leads to renal failure.

Nervous system Neurological involvement appears to be relatively uncommon in systemic sclerosis, but carpal tunnel syndrome and trigeminal neuropathy have been reported as associated abnormalities.

Cardiac Myocardial fibrosis, conduction disorders and a variety of ECG abnormalities have been described in systemic sclerosis.

Hepatic There is a significant association between systemic sclerosis and primary biliary cirrhosis.

Musculoskeletal Arthralgia and arthritis occur in some patients with systemic sclerosis. Myopathy and inflammatory myositis may also occur.

Treatment

Systemic steroid therapy is of no benefit in the majority of cases of systemic sclerosis, although steroids may be of help in patients with an inflammatory myositis. Penicillamine therapy is also usually ineffective. Digital ischaemia may be helped by wearing electrically heated gloves and socks. Prostacyclins, ketanserin or nifedipine may help relieve Raynaud's phenomenon. Patients with symptoms of oesophageal reflux should avoid lying flat, and may benefit from treatment with antacids, cimetidine and metoclopramide. Treatment with a broad-spectrum antibiotic such as a tetracycline may help patients with malabsorption secondary to bacterial overgrowth in the small bowel.

Prognosis

Severe pulmonary or renal involvement are poor prognostic factors, but the majority of patients suffering from systemic sclerosis live for many years.

Chemically-induced scleroderma

Polyvinyl chloride (PVC) can induce a disorder resembling idiopathic systemic sclerosis, and 'vinyl chloride disease' has been described in workers in the PVC industry, particularly reactor cleaners. A number of other chemicals may induce diseases mimicking systemic sclerosis, including perchlorethylene and trichlorethylene (solvents used in dry-cleaning), and bleomycin. A disorder similar to systemic sclerosis occurred in 1981 in a large number of people poisoned by ingestion of contaminated rape-seed oil sold as cooking oil in Madrid. The exact cause of this 'toxic oil syndrome' has yet to be established.

Pseudoscleroderma

Scleroderma-like changes may be seen in a number of conditions other than morphoea and systemic sclerosis. These include porphyria cutanea tarda, carcinoid syndrome, and phenylketonuria.

Chapter 18
Pruritus

There was a young belle of old Natchez
Whose garments were always in patches
When comment arose
On the state of her clothes
She drawled: 'When Ah itchez, Ah scratchez!'
(Ogden Nash, *Requiem*)

Pruritus means itching. Please note the correct spelling of the word: it is *not* spelt pruritis as it so often appears in student exam papers, clinical notes and referral letters! Pruritus may be of many different characters. Everyone has experienced short-term, localized itch and there is often a perverse joy in having a really good scratch. However, some people do not find pruritus any fun at all and suffer chronic irritation which may last for many years. Itching may be restricted to one or more sites, or it may cover virtually the whole of the body surface. Itch may creep about, appearing first on an arm and later on the back or in more than one site simultaneously. Itching can be mild and merely a nuisance or it can be appallingly severe, constant and distressing. Chronic pruritus can completely ruin the quality of life.

Pruritus is a prominent feature of many skin diseases, but not all. Especially itchy are the eczemas, lichen planus, insect bites and infestations, urticaria and dermatitis herpetiformis. However, the skin may also itch when there is no apparent cutaneous abnormality visible.

Mechanisms of pruritus

We do not clearly understand the mechanism of itching in inflammatory dermatoses, but at least there is a pathological process present, whose treatment may result in an improvement in symptoms. We understand even less well the phenomenon of irritation in otherwise apparently normal skin.

As with other modalities of cutaneous sensation, itch is probably produced, conditioned and appreciated by factors at all levels in the nervous system from stimulus, mediators and receptors via peripheral pathways to central processing and interpretation. It has been shown, for example, that a variety of stimuli can induce itch: pressure with a fine probe, electrical stimulation, heat and a number of chemicals. Important amongst these latter are histamine and a number of proteinases. Prostaglandins also enhance the itch sensation. It is not clear whether such agents act alone, or induce itch by stimulating the release of other chemicals. Even the role of histamine in itching remains obscure. It is known that histamine can induce itch even without wealing and can stimulate nerve endings directly, but non-sedative antihistamines generally have little effect on simple pruritus.

It is interesting that in experimental conditions, itching was found to be maximal when the stimulus was applied at the dermoepidermal junction. Many of the itchiest skin diseases have changes at the dermoepidermal junction. However, so do some of those in which itch is not such a prominent feature.

More complex, central mechanisms also seem to be important in the modulation and appreciation of pruritus. It is interesting that many of the stimuli which produce itch also induce pain if applied at higher intensities. Furthermore, the response of scratching the skin appears to induce pain in order to abolish irritation. However, other sensory stimuli such as pressure and vibration can also abolish itching and for these reasons a more complex mechanism for itch and its perception has to be sought. One such is the 'gate-control' theory. This proposes that a complicated segmental filtering system exists which opens and closes the input pathways to further stimuli as well as passing information on up to higher centres.

There is no doubt, too, that the sensation of itch can be modulated by higher centres themselves. Itch is much less apparent when the mind is fully occupied and much worse when boredom sets in, and there is no doubt that 'stress' and other psychological factors can induce or worsen pruritus. However, there is as yet no clear understanding of how such factors influence any sensation let alone one as capricious as pruritus.

Causes of pruritus

The term pruritus, when used without qualification, is often used to imply that there is itching without a primary skin disorder. However, it is important to note that in many instances there are considerable secondary skin changes from scratching such as excoriations, scars and prurigo (see below). A primary skin disorder, in which the changes are subtle, can easily be obscured by the results of the itching and scratching. The classical example of this is scabies (see Chapter 5). A full history and a careful examination of the skin is therefore important in all patients complaining of itching.

In considering the causes of pruritus, it is useful to look separately at those patients in whom the symptom is localized, those with a more generalized problem, and those with so-called 'senile' pruritus.

Localized pruritus

Localized irritation of the skin is common. On clinical examination, the skin may be otherwise apparently normal, but it is more common to find some abnormalities present. It is always important to try and exclude a primary cause for such changes because itching of localized areas of skin may, of course, be due to inflammatory skin disorders such as eczema (see Chapter 7) or dermatitis herpetiformis (see Chapter 14). It may also occur in patients with infestations such as scabies, head lice, pubic lice or where there are insects or mites in the domestic environment (see Chapter 5).

Two very important and troublesome forms of localized pruritus are lichen simplex chronicus and prurigo, and anogenital pruritus.

Lichen simplex chronicus and prurigo

This is a particularly difficult problem, which is sometimes labelled 'neuroder-matitis'. A state of constant irritation leads to constant scratching which, in turn, leads to thickening of the skin. This may occur in plaques, known as lichen simplex chronicus (Fig. 18.1) or in nodules, which are given the name 'prurigo' (Fig. 18.2). These areas of thickening are themselves irritable and an itch/scratch cycle is set up which becomes self-perpetuating.

Lichen simplex chronicus tends to affect certain classical sites, including the shins, the forearms, palms of the hands and the back of the neck (where the process is sometimes known as lichen nuchae). It may also involve perianal and vulval skin (see below). Prurigo nodules may accompany areas of lichen simplex or they may appear separately almost anywhere. They may be multiple.

The mechanisms involved in this process remain a mystery, although it is often suggested that patients who develop this kind of localized itching are rather tense. The diagnosis should be suspected when a thickened, assymmet-rical area of skin is intensely itchy and fails to respond satisfactorily to topical steroids alone. Some patients with lichen simplex chronicus can be improved by

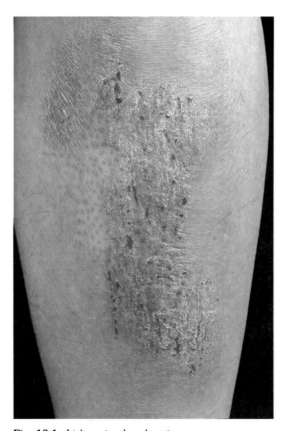

Fig. 18.1. Lichen simplex chronicus.

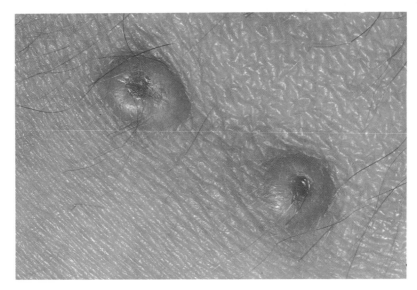

Fig. 18.2. Nodular prurigo.

using potent topical steroids under occlusive bandages impregnated with tar, but the problem often recurs.

Anogenital pruritus

Two of the most common (and least talked about) forms of localized itching are pruritus vulvae and pruritus ani.

Many doctors readily ascribe diagnoses to itch in the perineum quite erroneously. It is often assumed, for example, that perianal irritation is 'due to piles'. However, while haemorrhoids or skin tags are often found on examination, their treatment alone does not always relieve the symptoms. Another pitfall is to consider the problem to be wholly psychological. There may be psychological factors but only rarely are these the complete explanation. It is also very important that the patient is examined carefully for signs of cutaneous disease and inflammation, otherwise many important conditions will be missed.

Anal itching is not usually a prominent symptom until the late 20s but once it has begun it may continue for many years. The irritation is often spasmodic and extremely intense. The majority of patients are male.

Examination in many patients reveals relatively little. There may be some evidence of excoriation and some thickening of the anal and perianal skin, and there are often 'tags' present. However, these are also present in patients who do not suffer with anal itch. Occasionally there are gross changes amounting to lichen simplex secondary to scratching and there may be an associated fissure. Psoriasis of the natal cleft and perineum may give rise to pruritus ani.

The aetiology of this disorder is unknown but it is thought that the majority of instances of pruritus ani are essentially due to a low-grade irritant reaction to faeces, sweat and discharge. This is made worse by sedentary occupations.

Pruritus vulvae can be a very distressing symptom and there are a number of causes. Minor degrees of incontinence associated with prolapse may give rise to a similar irritant dermatitis to that seen in perianal itch. Several skin disorders may affect the vulva, notably ezcema and psoriasis, which are invariably itchy when they do. Lichen sclerosus et atrophicus has a predilection for the vulva and is a major cause of genital irritation (see Chapter 15). It is often mislabelled as 'leukoplakia'.

Some patients also develop allergic contact dermatitis to medicaments applied to the anogenital area. The topical anaesthetics cinchocaine, amethocaine, amylocaine, benzocaine and procaine are all potent sensitizers and many topical preparations for perineal itch contain one or more of them. This complication may also arise from preservatives or from other active constituents, especially antibiotics of the aminoglycoside family.

It also is important to remember that anogenital pruritus may be due to candidosis secondary to diabetes mellitus. The vulva is usually a beefy red, and there may be few pustules. Urine and blood sugar examination, together with perineal swabs should always be arranged if this is a possibility, especially in an elderly patient. If the diagnosis is confirmed, the itching will respond to topical anticandidal therapy with nystatin or an imidazole as long as the diabetes is also brought under control.

Finally, there are some instances in which pruritus vulvae et ani presents with no visible cutaneous abnormality at all and a true psychogenic origin is suspected. These patients seldom respond to simple antipruritic remedies and inexpert psychological probing is valueless. However, this is a diagnosis that should only be considered when all others have been excluded.

The management of anogenital itch depends upon its cause. Good hygiene and a high-fibre diet is recommended for the simple irritant type of pruritus ani. Treatment of any concomitant haemorrhoids may reduce discharge and improve matters somewhat, but the condition often continues in spite of this. For simple anogenital itch, where no other cause has been demonstrated, an initial course of powerful topical steroids should be followed by a gradual reduction in potency until the weakest effective preparation is found. For eczema, psoriasis, lichen sclerosus and other primary disorders the treatment will also consist largely of topical steroids, perhaps with some tar for psoriasis. A careful watch must be maintained in anyone with lichen sclerosus et atrophicus because there is a well-recognized risk of malignant change.

Generalized pruritus

Generalized pruritus is an extremely unpleasant symptom. The term is used to describe itching of a widespread character, which either continuously affects most of the body surface or involves several different areas, but in whom a primary skin disorder has been excluded.

The skin changes present in patients with generalized pruritus vary considerably. There may be nothing to see at all, there may be mild flakiness of the skin, with a few scratch marks, or the skin may be covered in excoriations, scars and nodules. The skin is often dry, especially in the elderly.

Although there may be no identifiable underlying disorder, all patients with generalized irritation of this kind should be investigated because there are a number of potentially remediable systemic disorders that may be responsible:

Haematological disorders
    Iron deficiency
    Polycythaemia rubra vera
Cholestatic liver disease
    Extrahepatic obstruction
    Primary biliary cirrhosis
    Hepatitis
    Drug-induced cholestasis
Chronic renal failure
Thyroid disease
    Thyrotoxicosis
    Myxoedema
Malignancy
    Lymphomas and leukaemias
    Carcinomas
Drug ingestion
    Opiates
Pregnancy
    (see Chapter 15)

Haematological disorders may present with generalized pruritus. Chronic iron deficiency may present in this way. This may be due to blood loss, for example from menorrhagia or a gut carcinoma. Many elderly patients are marginally or quite severely iron deficient for dietary reasons and so are some other groups, such as Hindu vegans. It is also well-known that pruritus may accompany polycythaemia rubra vera. This is often triggered by bathing. Such a history should immediately alert one to this possibility, although there is also a group of patients who itch after bathing but who have no haematological disorder. This is called aquagenic pruritus.

Irritation is a prominent feature of *liver disease*. The precise cause is unknown but it has been suggested that it is related to high bile salt concentrations in the skin. The main types of liver disease associated with itching have been outlined above. It is important to note that irritation may precede the development of other features of cholestatic liver disease, especially in primary biliary cirrhosis.

Chronic renal failure is becoming a more important cause of intractable pruritus because it is unfortunately largely unaffected by haemodialysis or peritoneal dialysis. As more and more patients are treated with these techniques, so more face the misery of chronic itch. Interestingly, parathyroidectomy can relieve the itch of chronic renal failure, but the action is generally short-lived and is hardly justified in most patients.

Thyroid disease certainly presents with pruritus, and both thyrotoxicosis and myxoedema may do so. The itch in myxoedema may be related to the general dryness of the skin which is seen in these patients.

Underlying *neoplasia* is also capable of inducing generalized pruritus. This may be a carcinoma but lymphoreticular malignancies are more commonly associated with this symptom. Up to 30% of patients with Hodgkin's disease suffer from generalized pruritus at some point in their illness. Patients with this and other lymphomas may present in this way, and, as with cholestasis, itching may precede the development of other features by some months.

Drugs of various kinds may also induce itching. The mechanisms involved are often not clearly understood, although opiates appear to act both on central pathways and on mast cells while others, such as oestrogens and phenothiazines induce cholestasis.

Diabetes mellitus is frequently quoted as a cause of generalized pruritus, but we would never be satisfied with this as an explanation unless all others had been excluded first. Diabetes often co-exists, for example, with renal disease. As mentioned above diabetes may present with anogenital irritation due to candidosis.

There is, however, no doubt that occasionally generalized pruritus may be attributable to *psychological factors*, usually an anxiety neurosis. Patients with monodelusional psychoses such as parasitophobia also itch, but they offer their own explanation only too readily! The relationship between the skin and the psyche is considered in Chapter 20.

It is not difficult to devise a simple set of screening tests to try to ensure that none of these systemic causes of generalized pruritus is missed: a full history and general examination, full blood count, ESR, liver function tests, blood urea, serum iron, serum thyroxine, urine protein and a chest X-ray. If excluding diabetes is important, we would recommend a blood sugar rather than a urine examination alone, as urinary thresholds may be misleading. It is important that these tests are repeated, if negative initially, and if the pruritus persists. Treatment of generalized pruritus is that of its cause. When no apparent underlying reason can be found, it is worth trying a topical steroid and a sedative antihistamine, such as hydroxyzine.

Senile pruritus and xerosis

A significant number of people develop itching as they get older. The symptoms usually appear in the 70s and beyond. The irritation may be mild and localized, but in some it is very severe and generalized. There is no obvious skin disease, investigation reveals no underlying disorder and, although they are often anxious and miserable, this is usually secondary to the irritation rather than a primary cause. It is these patients to whom the term senile pruritus, is generally applied. Examination of the skin divides them broadly into two groups: those where there is no apparent change apart from secondary scratch marks and those where there is surface dryness (or 'xerosis').

It is not known what causes apparently normal, but ageing, skin to itch and treatment is extremely difficult indeed. Sedative antihistamines often cause excessive drowsiness and confusion in the elderly, and topical steroids are of limited use. It may be helpful to use some of the measures which help senile xerosis (see below).

Dryness or roughness of the skin is very common in the elderly and many different terms have been used: 'pruritus hiemalis', 'prurigo hiemalis', 'winter eczema'. These simply reflect different facets of the condition. It is not at all clear why the skin becomes dry in old age.

It is apparently not due to an increase in water loss as is sometimes stated and there is no evidence that sebaceous gland dysfunction plays a role.

The process is not always generalized, but favours the lower legs, and is made worse by climatic and atmospheric conditions. In its most severe form (also known as 'eczema cracquelé' or 'asteatotic eczema') the skin becomes frankly inflamed as well as dry, resulting in a crazy-paving effect (see Chapter 7). This situation is most frequently encountered in centrally heated homes and hospital wards where the elderly often pass their final years.

The management of the xerosis of old age rests on the manipulation of the environment, if this is feasible, and effective use of emollients. The main environmental factors that are important are atmospheric humidity, together with temperature, and cutaneous contact with soaps, cleansers and other irritants. It is a common observation that cutaneous xerosis in the elderly is much worse in the winter (hence 'pruritus heimalis'; 'winter eczema'). The widespread use of central heating exaggerates this tendency.

An increase in the frequency of washing or the use of harsh soaps and detergents make matters worse, partly by removing surface lipids and partly by acting as direct irritants. Many irritant chemicals probably remain in ageing skin far longer than in young skin and, consequently, cause more damage. The atmosphere should be humidified if possible, and liberal quantities of emollient applied to the skin surface. Soaps should be discouraged as far as possible and use should be made of emollients instead. We recommend a simple bathing regime for those who can manage it:

Before the bath
    All-over application of emollient
In the bath
    Proprietary bath oil
    Non-soap cleanser
After the bath
    All-over application of emollient while skin is slightly damp

In general, the heavier the emollient, the better it will work. The bath will become very slippery and the elderly must be warned to take great care getting in and out. It is a good idea to use a non-slip mat. If bathing is difficult, the same general principles apply to the use of emollients but their application will have to be made as and when possible.

Chapter 19
Systemic Disease and the Skin

The skin may be involved directly or indirectly in a number of systemic disease processes, and provide visible diagnostic clues leading to the discovery of internal disease.

Endocrine disease

Diabetes

There are a number of cutaneous manifestations of diabetes, including:
1 Certain cutaneous infections.
2 Neuropathic ulcers.
3 Necrobiosis lipoidica diabeticorum.
3 Diabetic dermopathy.
5 Bullosis diabeticorum.
6 Xanthomas.
7 Effects of insulin injections on the skin and subcutaneous tissues.

1 *Cutaneous infection* Mucosal candidiasis, particularly balanitis and vulvo-vaginitis, tinea (pityriasis) versicolor, and staphylococcal carbuncles, occur more frequently in diabetics.

2 *Neuropathic ulcers* Impaired sensation, as a result of sensory neuropathy, predisposes to the development of neuropathic ulcers on the soles of the feet (Fig. 19.1).

3 *Necrobiosis lipoidica diabeticorum* The skin of the shins is the character-istic site for lesions of necrobiosis lipoidica, although they may occur on other parts of the body. The lesions are yellowish brown in colour, and atrophic, so that underlying small blood vessels are easily seen through the thinned skin (Fig. 19.2). Occasionally the lesions ulcerate. Not all patients with necrobiosis lipoidica are diabetic (approximately 50% presenting with the skin lesions), and of the others, some will subsequently develop diabetes. Good diabetic control does not appear to influence the skin lesions.

Topical and intralesional steroids are used in the treatment of necrobiosis lipoidica, but results of treatment are not very impressive.

4 *Diabetic dermopathy* The term diabetic dermopathy is applied to small, brown, scar-like lesions seen on the shins in some diabetics. The lesions are apparently associated with diabetic microangiopathy.

5 *Bullosis diabeticorum* In this uncommon blistering disorder of diabetics subepidermal bullae occur on the hands and feet, without any obvious pre-existing inflammatory change. The aetiology of these blisters is unknown.

6 *Xanthomas* Hyperlipidaemia in uncontrolled diabetes may be associated with the development of multiple small, yellow eruptive xanthomas on trunk and limbs.

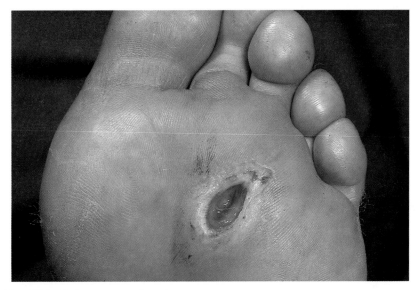

Fig. 19.1. Diabetic neuropathic ulcer.

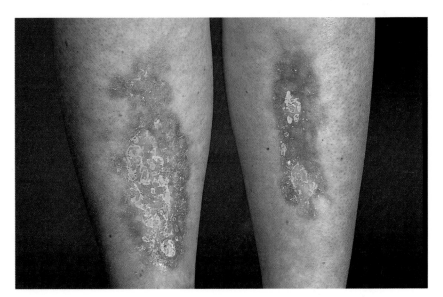

Fig. 19.2. Necrobiosis lipoidica diabeticorum.

7 *Effects of insulin injections* Insulin injections may cause lipoatrophy or fat hypertrophy ('insulin tumours') at injection sites.

Miscellaneous
  Other cutaneous manifestations include acanthosis nigricans in association with insulin-resistant diabetes, insulin-resistant diabetes associated with partial or

generalized cutaneous lipoatrophy, and a scleroderma-like thickening of the skin of the hands (diabetic acrosclerosis) in insulin-dependent diabetics.

Granuloma annulare   There is no significant association between classical granuloma annulare and diabetes, but in the much rarer generalized form of granuloma annulare there is a high incidence of diabetes. Typically, lesions of granuloma annulare are groups of firm, skin-coloured papules, often arranged in rings, and commonly occurring on the dorsa of the hands and feet (Fig. 19.3). The natural history of granuloma annulare is eventual spontaneous resolution, but persistent lesions may be treated with potent topical steroids or intralesional triamcinolone.

Thyroid disease

Hypothyroidism

In hypothroidism the skin is typically dry, and feels thickened due to subcutaneous mucin deposition—hence the designation myxoedema. A malar flush on an otherwise pale visage produces what has been referred to as a 'strawberries and cream' appearance. There may be a yellowish tinge to the skin, said to be due to the deposition of carotenes. There is often peri-orbital oedema. The scalp hair is coarse and brittle, and there is loss of the outer part of the eyebrows. Huddling close to the fire to keep warm may lead to severe erythema ab igne ('granny's tartan') on the shins.

Hyperthyroidism

Cutaneous changes which may accompany thyrotoxicosis include hyperhidrosis, palmar erythema, diffuse scalp alopecia, generalized hyperpigmentation,

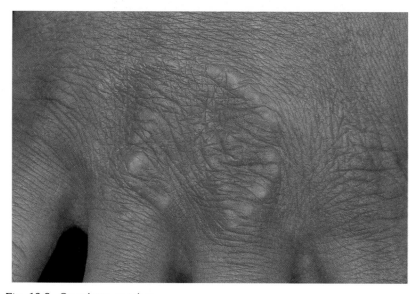

Fig. 19.3. Granuloma annulare.

and thyrotoxic acropachy (digital clubbing). The nails may show onycholysis. Patients with high circulating levels of long-acting thyroid stimulator (LATS) may develop pretibial myxoedema, which is produced by subcutaneous deposition of excessive amounts of mucopolysaccharide, usually over the shins and dorsa of the feet (Fig. 19.4). Plaques of pretibial myxoedema have an inflammatory appearance initially, and subsequently develop a rugose and verrucous surface.

Vitiligo may accompany autoimmune thyroid disease, and generalized pruritus may be a feature of both hypo- and hyperthyroidism.

Adrenal disease

Cushing's syndrome The cutaneous effects of Cushing's syndrome include thinning of the skin, spontaneous bruising, prominent purple striae on the trunk and limbs, diffuse alopecia, acne and hirsutism.

Addison's disease Diffuse hyperpigmentation is the main cutaneous manifestation of Addison's disease. The pigmentation is particularly prominent on the

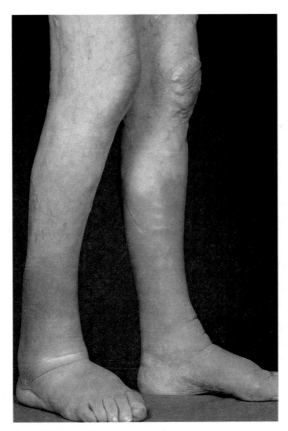

Fig. 19.4. Pretibial myxoedema.

buccal mucosa and in the palmar creases. Vitiligo may also accompany autoimmune Addison's disease.

Rheumatic diseases

Gout

In addition to tophaceous deposits around affected joints, gouty tophi may occur on the ears.

Still's disease (systemic juvenile chronic arthritis)

This is a disorder of childhood, although it may rarely occur in adults. Accompanying the pyrexial episodes of Still's disease is a diffuse maculopapular eruption which characteristically develops in the late afternoon and evening, and usually resolves by the following morning, only to reappear later in the day. Some slander-mongers claim that dermatologists never see this eruption because its periodicity is outside their normal working day.

Rheumatoid arthritis

Dermatological features of rheumatoid arthritis include:

1 *Rheumatoid nodules* Subcutaneous nodules over bony prominences, particularly on the extensor aspect of the forearms and the dorsa of the hands.
2 *Vasculitic lesions* Digital vasculitis may produce small infarcts around the nail folds (Bywaters' lesions), or more severe digital ulceration and even gangrene. Vasculitic lesions may also occur on the legs, and contribute to the formation of leg ulcers.
3 *Pyoderma gangrenosum.*
4 *Palmar erythema.*

Rheumatic fever

Almost extinct in developed countries, rheumatic fever may be accompanied by a characteristic eruption, erythema marginatum.

Reiter's syndrome

Predominantly a disease of young adult males, Reiter's syndrome is usually precipitated by non-specific urethritis, but occasionally by bacillary dysentery. In addition to urethritis, conjunctivitis/uveitis, and arthritis, there may be an eruption which is indistinguishable from psoriasis. On the soles of the feet the skin lesions may become extremely thickened producing so-called 'keratoderma blenorrhagica'. For some strange reason keratoderma blenorrhagica is a name which doctors in training always seem to be able to remember, probably because of the effort required to learn such bizarre terminology—it would be much easier to remember 'thick psoriasis'. The buccal mucosa may show scattered erosions, and superficial circumferential erosive changes on the penis are referred to as 'circinate balanitis'.

Vitamin deficiency

Scurvy

The classical picture of vitamin C (ascorbic acid) deficiency is rarely seen nowadays in developed countries, but scurvy may be encountered in the elderly and in alcoholics, as a result of nutritional self-neglect. The typical appearance is of perifollicular purpura, easy bruising, poor wound healing, bleeding gums, and woody oedema of the legs. The diagnosis can be confirmed by estimating leukocyte ascorbic acid levels.

Pellagra

This is a disorder resulting from nicotinic acid deficiency. Classically, pellagra has three major manifestations, dermatitis, diarrhoea and dementia—the so-called '3-D's'. The dermatitis affects light-exposed areas, and there is often a well-demarcated margin to the affected area on the neck (Casal's necklace). Pellagra may occur in alcoholics as a result of nutritional self-neglect. A similar dermatitis may be provoked by isoniazid in individuals who are slow acetylators of this drug, and who also have low dietary intake of vitamins.

Inflammatory bowel disease

Ulcerative colitis and Crohn's disease may be associated with a number of mucocutaneous manifestations including:

1 *Pyoderma gangrenosum* The pathological basis of lesions of pyoderma gangrenosum is probably a vasculitis. The lesions may be single or multiple, and initially resemble boils which break down to form necrotic ulcers with overhanging purple edges (Fig. 19.5). Pyoderma gangrenosum may also occur in association with rheumatoid arthritis, multiple myeloma and leukaemia. The

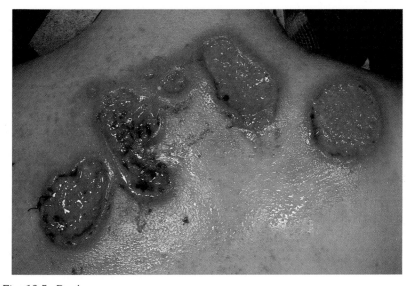

Fig. 19.5. Pyoderma gangrenosum.

treatment of choice is systemic steroids, but pyoderma gangrenosum may also respond to azathioprine, minocycline or clofazimine.

2 *Erythema nodosum.*

3 *Perianal and buccal mucosal lesions* May accompany Crohn's disease. Anal examination may reveal fleshy tags, fissures, and perianal fistulae. The buccal mucosa may be oedematous and ulcerated, and the lips may be swollen as a result of a granulomatous cheilitis.

Hyperlipidaemia

Both primary and secondary hyperlipidaemic states may be associated with lipid deposits in the skin, known as xanthomas. There are several different clinical types of xanthomas. Orange-yellow lipid deposits in the eyelid skin are known as xanthelasma (Fig. 19.6). Only a proportion of patients with xanthelasma have a demonstrable elevation of plasma lipids. Tuberous xanthomas occur as yellowish nodules, often on the knees and elbows (Fig. 19.7). Tendinous xanthomas, as their name suggests, are deposits of lipid in association with tendons, often involving the Achilles tendons and extensor tendons on the dorsa of the hands. Deposits of lipid in the skin creases of the hands (xanthoma striatum palmare) appear to be particularly associated with primary Type III hyperlipidaemia. Eruptive xanthomas are crops of yellowish papules which occur in association with marked hypertriglyceridaemia.

Amyloidosis

In systemic amyloidosis, amyloid deposits in the tongue produce macroglossia, and cutaneous deposits are visible as yellowish, waxy, purpuric plaques around the eyes and in the perianal area.

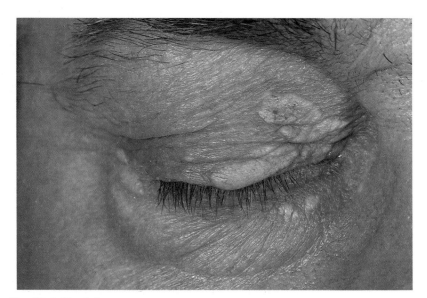

Fig. 19.6. Xanthelasma.

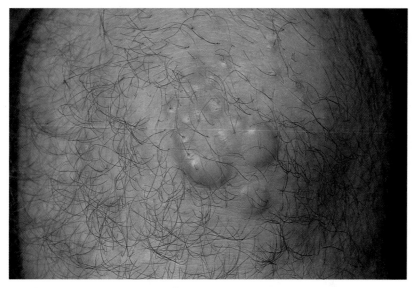

Fig. 19.7. Tuberous xanthomas.

Sarcoidosis

Sarcoidosis is a multisystem granulomatous disorder of unknown aetiology. There are a number of patterns of skin involvement in sarcoidosis, including:

1 *Erythema nodosum* These tender, erythematous nodules on the legs are the result of a panniculitis (*see* Chapter 16). One of the commonest presentations of sarcoidosis is the 'erythema nodosum—arthropathy—bilateral hilar lymphadenopathy syndrome'.

2 *Lupus pernio* The skin of the nose and ears becomes infiltrated with granulomas, swollen and purplish in colour.

3 *Scar sarcoid* Sarcoid granulomas localize in old scar tissue, making the scars particularly prominent.

4 *Papules, nodules and plaques* Often with an orange-brown colour. Plaques may be psoriasiform in appearance.

Liver disease and the skin

Changes in the skin and nails occurring in association with chronic liver disease include:

1 Palmar erythema.

2 Pruritus: in cholestatic liver disease.

3 Spider naevi: in a superior vena caval distribution.

4 Xanthelasma: in primary biliary cirrhosis.

5 White nails (Terry's nails).

6 Pigmentary changes: in addition to jaundice, patients with long-standing cholestatic liver disease may also have marked melanin pigmentation. Patients suffering from haemochromatosis have generalized bronze-brown hyperpigmentation which is produced by a melanin.

Cutaneous manifestations of systemic malignancy

Cutaneous metastases

Malignant tumours may metastasize to the skin, and tumours of renal, ovarian, gastrointestinal, breast and bronchial origin are those most likely to do so (Fig. 19.8). Cutaneous metastases usually appear as nondescript pink nodules, and they are sited most frequently on the scalp and anterior trunk. Scalp secondaries may produce areas of alopecia (alopecia neoplastica).

Lymphatic extension of carcinoma to the skin may produce an area of inflammatory induration resembling cellulitis known as 'carcinoma erysipelatoides'.

Metastasis of ovarian or gastrointestinal carcinoma via the ligamentum teres can present as an umbilical nodule (Sister Joseph's nodule).

Miscellaneous cutaneous signs of underlying malignancy

1   *Dermatomyositis* (see Chapter 17).

2   *Acanthosis nigricans* This is a warty, hyperpigmented thickening of the skin in the axillae and groins (Fig. 19.9). The palms of the hands may also be affected, giving an appearance known as 'tripe palms'. The commonest associated malignancy is an adenocarcinoma of the gastrointestinal tract. Remember, however, that 'malignant' acanthosis nigricans is relatively rare, whereas flexural acanthosis nigricans is extremely common in the obese and is unrelated to systemic problems.

3   *Generalized pruritus* Generalized itching may be associated with a wide variety of systemic malignancies.

4   *Thrombophlebitis migrans* This is particularly associated with carcinoma of the pancreas.

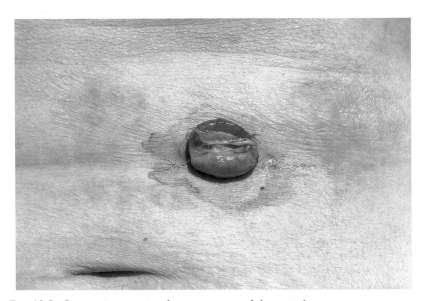

Fig. 19.8. Cutaneous metastasis from carcinoma of the oesophagus.

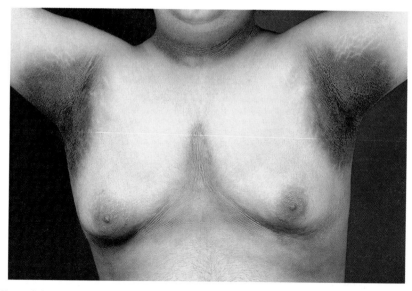

Fig. 19.9. Acanthosis nigricans.

5 *Acquired ichthyosis* Ichthyosis developing for the first time in adult life may be associated with a lymphoma.

6 *Bullous pemphigoid* (see Chapter 14).

7 *Erythema multiforme* An erythema multiforme-like eruption may accompany systemic neoplasia.

8 *The sign of Leser Trélat* This is the sudden development of a profusion of seborrhoeic warts, as a manifestation of systemic malignancy.

9 *Bullous pyoderma gangrenosum* May occur with leukaemia and myeloma.

10 *Acquired hypertrichosis lanuginosa* The sudden growth of profuse vellus hair over the face and body is a rare sign of underlying neoplastic disease.

11 *Necrolytic migratory erythema* This is a distinctive eruption associated with a pancreatic glucagonoma.

12 *Flushing* and a rosacea-like facial eruption are cutaneous features of the carcinoid syndrome.

13 *Erythema gyratum repens* This rare skin marker of malignancy is a bizarre patterned erythema resembling 'wood grain'.

Leukaemia and the skin

There are numerous cutaneous changes which may accompany leukaemia, and be provoked by the drugs used in its treatment.

Common presenting features of acute leukaemia include purpura, bruising, and bleeding from the gums, and leukaemia may involve the skin directly in the form of leukaemic infiltrates. Disseminated herpes zoster, i.e. herpes zoster with numerous outlying vesicles, may accompany leukaemia, as may a severe bullous form of pyoderma gangrenosum, and Sweet's disease (acute febrile neutrophilic dermatosis).

Bone marrow transplantation

Graft-versus-host reactions (GVHR) following bone marrow transplantation affect the skin, liver and gut. The earliest sign of GVHR in the skin, usually occurring within 2–3 weeks of the transplant if it has engrafted, is a morbilliform (measles-like) eruption accompanied by erythema of the hands and feet. Occasionally these changes are very florid and progress to toxic epidermal necrolysis (see Chapter 14). In chronic graft-versus-host reactions changes occur in the skin and buccal mucosa which are clinically identical to those seen in lichen planus (see Chapter 15). A later manifestation of chronic GVHR is the development of scleroderma-like changes in the skin (see Chapter 17).

Purpura

Purpura is produced by extravasation of red cells into the skin, and has numerous causes. The lesions of purpura do not blanch on pressure.

Causes of purpura include vasculitis (see Chapter 16), quantitative or qualitative platelet abnormalities, certain drugs (e.g. carbromal), amyloidosis, dysproteinaemias, and infections (e.g. meningococcaemia).

AIDS and the skin

Patients suffering from the Acquired Immunodeficiency Syndrome (AIDS), caused by the Human Immunodeficiency Virus (HIV), are at increased risk of developing a number of mucocutaneous problems, including:

1 Oral candidiasis and Candida intertrigo.

2 Oral 'hairy leukoplakia': clinically this presents as ribbed white areas along the sides of the tongue. The appellation 'hairy' relates to the histological appearance of projections of keratinized squamous epithelium. There is evidence to suggest that human papilloma viruses and viruses of the herpes group play a part in producing hairy leukoplakia.

3 Gingivitis.

4 Seborrhoeic dermatitis: this is probably related to proliferation of, or altered response to, pityrosporum yeasts.

5 Itchy folliculitis: the aetiology of this non-specific pruritic folliculitis is unknown.

6 Shingles, molluscum contagiosum and dermatophyte fungal infections occur more commonly in AIDS patients.

7 Episodes of herpes simplex are more frequent and more severe.

8 Perianal warts tend to be more florid and more difficult to treat effectively.

9 Kaposi's sarcoma: Kaposi's sarcoma is a malignant tumour which is thought to arise from vascular endothelium, but its precise cell type of origin has not been established with certainty. In patients suffering from AIDS, lesions of Kaposi's sarcoma are usually multiple, and may affect any part of the skin, as well as internal organs. Kaposi's sarcoma is rarely the cause of death in AIDS patients, who usually succumb to intercurrent infection. It is a radiosensitive tumour.

Chapter 20
Skin and the Psyche

> If you happen to have a wart on your nose or forehead, you cannot help imagining that no
> one in the world has anything else to do but stare at your wart, laugh at it, and condemn
> you for it, even though you have discovered America.
>
> (Fyodor Dostoevsky, *The Idiot*)

A frequent question posed by patients during discussion of the aetiology of their skin disease is 'Is it caused by nerves doctor?' 'Nerves' is used as a sort of generic term in this context, but what the patient is usually trying to say is can he or she attribute the onset of the skin problem to a stressful situation. In fact, very few skin disorders are directly related to psychological disturbance, although sometimes 'nerves' seems a much simpler explanation to give to the patient than four words of inexplicable Latin mumbo jumbo describing a condition of unknown aetiology. There is certainly a great deal of anecdotal evidence that psoriasis and atopic eczema may be exacerbated by stress, but the pathomechanics of such an association are obscure and it is therefore difficult to confirm a direct cause and effect relationship. Other conditions in which emotional stress has been claimed to play a part in some cases include alopecia areata and acute pompholyx.

There is no doubt, however, that skin disease has psychological effects on the sufferer, and sometimes these are profound. Skin disease is visible to others, it carries the taint of contagion, and it is something which is socially unacceptable because of public ignorance and superstition. It requires considerable courage for an individual with a chronic dermatosis of the face or hands to work in an occupation which involves contact with the general public. They will be aware that their skin is being scrutinized and that any form of physical contact, such as shaking hands or collecting change, provokes apprehension. In certain ethnic groups where marriages are arranged, the presence of skin disease in one prospective partner may compromise their marriage prospects, and cause considerable emotional distress. Infestations with ectoparasites sometimes have marked psychological effects. Patients feel unclean, and these feelings can persist long after the problem has been eradicated.

There are some skin disorders which are directly related to psychological problems, and these include the following conditions:

Dermatitis artefacta

This is the dermatological equivalent of the Munchausen syndrome. It is part of a wide spectrum of factitious disease. Patients with dermatitis artefacta produce their skin lesions to satisfy a psychological need, but what benefit they derive from their actions is usually not obvious. They will vehemently deny that the lesions are self-induced if challenged. As a group they are distinct from

239

malingerers, who imitate or produce an illness for a deliberate end, and are quite conscious of what they are doing, and why they are doing it.

Artefactual skin lesions may be produced in a number of different ways including rubbing, scratching, picking, gouging, puncturing, cutting, sucking, biting, the application of heat or caustics, or the injection of milk, blood and faecal material (Fig. 20.1). Limb oedema may be simulated by the intermittent application of a tourniquet. The lesions produced by these methods tend to have bizarre geometric shapes which do not conform to natural disease—no dermatosis has square, rectangular or triangular lesions. Often the lesions are more numerous on the side of the body opposite the dominant hand. If a caustic material has been used to induce lesions this may trickle off the main area of damage to produce tell-tale streaks at the margins. Even when lesions suspected of being artefactual are covered by occlusive dressings, patients will often manage to insert knitting needles under the dressings, or push sharp instruments through them. This has led cunning physicians to devise techniques of detecting this interference by methods such as the inclusion of aluminium foil in the dressings so that perforation from outside can be detected.

The incidence of dermatitis artefacta is higher in women, and most of those affected are adolescents or young adults. It is also quite common to find that they have some connection with the health professions, either directly or via family members. The history obtained from these patients about their skin problem is devoid of any useful information about the evolution of their lesions. The impression conveyed is that one minute the skin was normal, and the next it was blemished. This 'hollow history' is characteristic of dermatitis artefacta. Another characteristic feature is a striking complacency about what are often extremely disfiguring lesions ('*la belle indifférence*'). The authors have encoun-

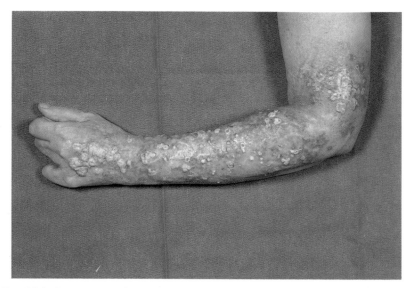

Fig. 20.1. Dermatitis artefacta—in this case probably the result of inoculation of faeces into the skin.

tered one patient with extensive suppuration of the left arm, probably produced by the inoculation of faeces, who said 'Yes, it is rather unpleasant isn't it, I wonder if you could arrange for someone to take it off.'

The psychopathology of patients who produce artefacts is not uniform. Some patients produce lesions to draw attention to other problems, or as part of a personality disorder. In others, dermatitis artefacta represents a hysterical conversion or other hysterical reaction.

It requires considerable expertise in dermatology to be able to make a confident diagnosis of dermatitis artefacta, but even the experienced dermatologist will see cases where he suspects artefact, but cannot be certain.

Treatment is difficult, if not impossible. Confronting the patient with the diagnosis usually produces a categorical denial, and subsequent failure to attend for follow-up. Attempts to strictly occlude the traumatized area may allow healing to occur, but the lesions will reappear as soon as occlusive dressings are removed. A rather more alarming result of occlusion may be the appearance of lesions elsewhere, or the development of other symptoms to compensate for the inability to reach the usual sites. Psychiatric referral is often unhelpful, and in many cases the patient will refuse the offer of assistance from a psychiatrist. With most patients the situation remains at stalemate. The dermatologist does not confront them with the diagnosis, and they continue to visit the dermatologist. It is probably a 'You know that I know that you know' situation, but as long as suspicions are not voiced it seems to suit the patients' needs, and they are quite happy to continue attending for follow-up.

The course of this disorder is often protracted. Recovery usually has nothing to do with successful medical treatment, but occurs because of increasing maturity, marriage, or having a family.

Dermatological pathomimicry

Dermatological pathomimicry is distinct from dermatitis artefacta. Patients with this syndrome either deliberately perpetuate their skin disease, or reproduce a pre-existing skin disorder. Having been appraised of the aetiology of their skin disease, they use this knowledge to reproduce the lesions when under emotional stress, to obtain sympathy, or in an effort to avoid an unpleasant situation with which they cannot cope. Examples of the type of illness used by patients for pathomimicry include allergic contact dermatitis, drug reactions, and chronic leg ulceration. This type of patient usually responds to positive direct psychotherapy.

Dermatological non-disease (dysmorphophobia)

In this condition patients complain of severe symptomatology localized to certain parts of the body, most commonly the face, scalp and perineum, but without any objective evidence of disease. The complaints include dysaesthesias such as burning, itching, or throbbing pain; too much or too little hair on the face or scalp, or altered texture of scalp hair; or the belief that they are the source of an offensive odour. These delusional beliefs or perceptions of abnormal sensations are a consuming preoccupation for the patient. A common presentation is a female patient complaining of a burning sensation in the perineum. She will already have seen a multiplicity of doctors, including several gynaecologists, and probably also surgeons, and will have undergone examination under anaesthetic, proctoscopy and sigmoidoscopy, all with negative results. The perineum looks completely normal, and *is* completely normal, but it does not *feel* completely normal to the patient.

In many cases depression is part of the clinical picture, and affected individuals may commit suicide. Untreated the condition will continue indefinitely, but some patients will respond to treatment with antidepressants and psychotherapy.

Delusions of parasitosis (parasitophobia: Ekbom's disease)

An experienced dermatologist will recognize cases of this condition from the referral letter, and will often arrange to see the patient at the end of a clinic, because the consultation is usually extremely lengthy. The typical parasitophobic is an anxious individual, often a middle-aged or elderly lady, who will already have consulted the local university Department of Zoology or museums to identify 'parasites', and will be well known to 'Rentokil' and the Environmental Health Department, who may have visited their home to 'disinfest' the premises. Members of the family may have been barred from visiting their home because of the risk of contagion, and they may have isolated themselves from friends and acquaintances because of their fear of passing the 'infestation', on to them. Because of their absolute conviction that they are infested they may have convinced their family, friends, and even their general practitioner of the reality of their problem (shared delusion).

Parasitophobics often describe a feeling of itching, biting or 'crawling' in the skin, and state that when this occurs they are able to remove a small 'insect' or 'worm' from a skin lesion. When asked to demonstrate typical skin lesions they will point to Campbell de Morgan spots, senile lentigines, etc., or even to perfectly normal skin where they imagine the lesions to be. Typical 'specimens' are presented to the doctor wrapped in bits of folded paper or adhesive tape, and kept in a match box. These should always be examined under the microscope, because they just might contain parasites, but usually they contain fragments of cotton, and skin debris.

It is impossible to persuade these patients that parasites are not responsible for their condition. If they are shown that their specimens are simple debris they remain unconvinced, and may even suggest that their parasites are so small that an electron microscope will be required to demonstrate them. In this situation the most lucid, eloquent discourse will fall upon deaf ears—the patient's beliefs remain unshaken, and the doctor retires from the conflict feeling more than somewhat jaded.

Delusions of parasitosis may occur in association with organic brain disease such as senile dementia and cerebral arteriosclerosis, but the majority of patients are said to fall into one of three diagnostic categories: paranoia; paranoid schizophrenia; or involutional depression in an individual whose premorbid personality was obsessive.

Effective treatment is difficult, and many parasitophobics continue with their delusions for years. Confrontation and explanation that they have a delusion rarely achieves anything. Parasitophobics often refuse psychiatric help because they do not accept that they have a mental illness, and cannot see how a psychiatrist could help with what to them is a physical disorder. However, if possible, they should be persuaded that a psychiatrist can help, because he has the expertise to treat the background psychopathology. The neuroleptic drug pimozide may be of benefit in parasitophobia, if one can persuade the patient to take it.

Obsessive-compulsive habits

Trichotillomania

Trichotillomania is a term applied to compulsive plucking of hair. The scalp is involved more frequently than other hair-bearing areas, but the eyebrows and eyelashes may be affected. A mild form of trichotillomania may be observed in medical libraries, where engrossed students compulsively twist locks of hair around their fingers, but rarely pluck it out unless finals are approaching. The clinical picture in trichotillomania is of patches of hair loss containing hairs of varying length. Often the crown of the head is affected and the hair at the margins of the scalp is of normal length (Fig. 20.2). The underlying scalp is usually normal, but may be excoriated.

Trichotillomania in childhood is often a transient compulsive habit. However, it may be a manifestation of disturbed behaviour or serious psychiatric illness, particularly in adults.

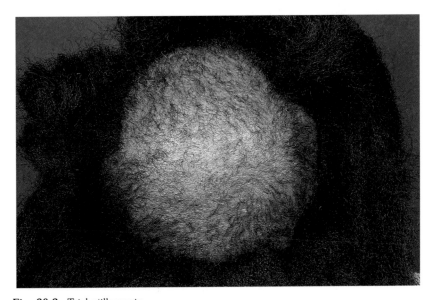

Fig. 20.2. Trichotillomania.

Neurotic excoriations

Neurotic excoriations are encountered much more frequently in women than in men. The lesions are produced by picking and gouging the skin, and are usually scattered over the arms, upper trunk and face. More recent lesions are usually interspersed with scars from previous excoriations. Acne excoriée is a variant of this condition in which minimal acne lesions are repeatedly picked and gouged with finger nails, leaving quite prominent scars when the lesions eventually heal.

Patients with this problem have obsessive-compulsive personalities, and picking the skin appears to provide relief of unconscious aggression and tension.

Chapter 21
Cutaneous Drug Reactions

There are only two types of drug—those that don't work and those that have side effects
(Bruno Handel FRCS)

The skin is one of the commonest sites for unwanted drug effects (a better term than 'side-effects'), although estimates of the frequency of such reactions vary considerably. Reactions to drugs are probably under-reported and often go unrecognized.

There is also no doubt that skin disorders that are not related to drug ingestion at all are labelled erroneously as cutaneous reactions to drugs. It is very important not to jump to conclusions. We have seen many common skin diseases such as herpes simplex, seborrhoeic dermatitis, acne, scabies, pityriasis rosea, pityriasis versicolor and chicken pox which have been cheerfully labelled as drug reactions. There are also undoubtedly a number of people who seem quite proud of being 'allergic to penicillin', who are no such thing.

It is also important to appreciate that there are currently no reliable *in vitro* tests for establishing that a skin change is due to a drug reaction. Simple *in vivo* tests, such as prick testing and patch testing, may have a limited place in specific situations, but yield no useful information in the majority of instances. It is important to stress that cutaneous drug reactions may be due to a variety of different mechanisms: simple intolerance, hypersensitivity reactions of Types I, II, III and IV, pharmacokinetic disturbances, drug interactions, complex interactions between host, drug and environment (e.g. light). Furthermore, even if the mechanism(s) were clearly known for a particular reaction, the chosen test might not be appropriate because the reaction is to a drug-complex or metabolite which occurs only *in vivo* after ingestion rather than to the original compound itself. The process of designing a set of tests to sort out any potential drug reaction must take all these factors into account.

The one truly definitive test available is a direct challenge of the patient with the suspected agent but it may be impossible or unethical to do this in many circumstances. It is, therefore, often not possible to prove categorically that a specific eruption was due to a specific drug and clinical judgements may have to be made on suspicion.

Drug reaction patterns

However, all is not lost! Some drugs are much more prone to induce cutaneous drug reaction patterns than others:

antibiotics, especially penicillin, semisynthetic penicillins and sulphonamides
non-steroidal anti-inflammatory drugs
hypnotics
tranquillizers

Furthermore, there are a number of well-defined clinical drug reaction patterns that can be recognized with experience:

Exanthematic eruptions
Urticaria and anaphylaxis
Exfoliative dermatitis
Vasculitis
Fixed drug eruptions
Lichen planus-like eruptions
Erythema multiforme
Acneiform eruptions
Hair abnormalities
Pigmentary changes
Bullous reactions
Photosensitivity
Lupus erythematosus-like syndrome
Exacerbation of pre-existing skin disease

We shall discuss these in a little more detail, highlighting the fact that these patterns may be more drug-specific and therefore recognition of them as drug reactions may help to isolate the culprit.

Exanthematic eruptions

These are the commonest cutaneous drug reactions of all. The rash, which is usually itchy, is widespread, symmetrical, erythematous and maculopapular (Fig. 21.1): it often strongly resembles a viral exanthem. The time relationship between the skin changes and the drug is variable. In most instances they begin within a few days of starting on the drug, but they may begin almost immediately, or be delayed for 2 or 3 weeks. Exanthematic eruptions usually fade over a period of a week or so after stopping the drug, but if the offending agent is not withdrawn, an exfoliative dermatitis (see below and Chapter 15) may develop.

The drugs most likely to provoke an exanthematic eruption are non-steroidal anti-inflammatory drugs and antibiotics, particularly ampicillin, other semisynthetic penicillins, sulphonamides and gentamicin. Rarer causes include gold, barbiturates and phenothiazines.

Urticaria and anaphylaxis (see also Chapter 15)

Urticaria is another skin reaction commonly triggered by drugs. It may be induced by a direct pharmacological action on mast cells (e.g. aspirin, opiates) or it may be due to a Type I or a Type III hypersensitivity reaction (e.g. pencillins, cephalosporins, pollen vaccines and toxoids).

Occasionally, the same group of drugs may trigger a major anaphylactic reaction, with or without urticaria. Such a reaction is often fatal unless treated very rapidly. Unfortunately, there is no known way of predicting this kind of disaster.

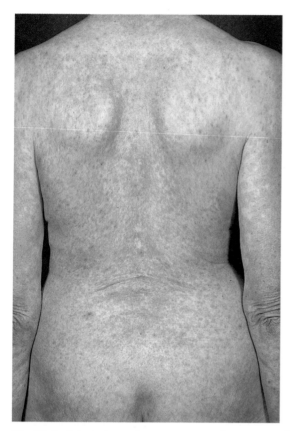

Fig. 21.1. A typical exanthematic eruption due to an antibiotic.

Eczema

Type IV hypersensitivity reactions to medicaments applied topically to the skin are common. Well-known examples include: lanolin in creams and bandages; preservatives (parabens, ethylenediamine) in creams; topical anaesthetics (not lignocaine); topical antihistamines; topical antibiotics, especially aminoglycosides, in creams and drops. The result of topical exposure to these agents in a sensitized individual is contact dermatitis (see Chapter 7). Fig 21.2 shows a woman who has been treated with eye drops containing an aminoglycoside antibiotic.

Occasionally, a patient may receive a compound systemically to which he or she has become sensitized by the topical route. The result is a widespread eczematous reaction, which can be very difficult to control. This most commonly occurs with an aminoglycoside (many cross-react), but aminophylline contains ethylenediamine and can also induce such a reaction.

Exfoliative dermatitis

Drugs are one the four important causes of exfoliative dermatitis (see Chapter 15). Many drugs have been reported in association with exfoliative dermatitis,

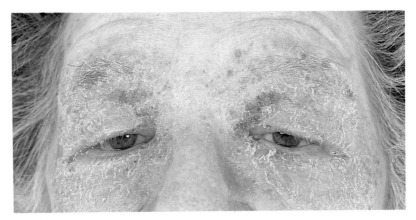

Fig. 21.2. Contact sensitivity to neomycin.

but prominent offenders are sulphonamides and sulphonylureas, gold, pheny-toin, allopurinol and barbiturates.

Vasculitis

Small-vessel inflammation due to the deposition of immune complexes may occur in a number of different clinical situations (see Chapter 16). However, one of the commonest causes is drug ingestion. The changes are most prominent on the lower legs, at least initially, and may vary from a few small pink and purpuric papules to quite large lesions with bullae or central necrosis. There may be renal involvement.

In our experience, thiazides are the drugs most frequently implicated in such reactions but vasculitis has also been reported with captopril, cimetidine, quinidine, sulphonamides and some others.

Fixed drug eruptions

Fixed drug eruptions are one of the most curious events encountered in dermatological practice. The reaction occurs in the same place(s) on each occasion that the offending drug is taken. They are often misdiagnosed by the unwary as recurrent eczema or ringworm.

The skin changes consist of a round or oval patch of dusky erythema, often with a purplish centre (Fig. 21.3). A central bulla sometimes forms. This fades to leave an area of postinflammatory hyperpigmentation. There may be only one such lesion, or the reaction may occur at multiple sites. Fixed eruptions can occur anywhere, although the limbs and genitalia are favoured sites.

Laxatives containing phenolphthalein, sulphonamides, dapsone, tetracy-clines, barbiturates and chlordiazipoxide have all been implicated in fixed drug eruptions.

Lichen planus-like eruptions

Although lichen planus-like (sometimes known as 'lichenoid') reactions are not very common, they can be severe. The eruption is occasionally indistinguishable

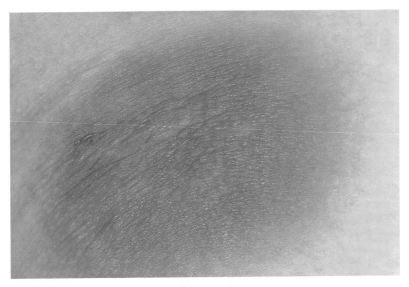

Fig. 21.3. Fixed drug reaction to a sulphonamide.

from idiopathic lichen planus. More commonly, although there is a resemblance, the eruption is more widespread, there are eczematous elements and there is much more scaling than is generally seen in lichen planus. The process may continue to progress, even after drug therapy is withdrawn. In severe cases this can result in an exfoliative dermatitis (see above and Chapter 15). Lichen planus-like drug reactions were first reported with antimalarial drugs, but are seen with some β-blockers and sulphonylureas. Gold is also an important cause, and thiazides may be associated with lichen planus-like eruptions on light-exposed surfaces.

Erythema multiforme (see Chapter 15)

It is not always easy to be certain whether a drug has provoked erythema multiforme. The reaction can be precipitated by a wide variety of infections and disease-states. However, it has been suggested that barbiturates, long-acting sulphonamides, cotrimoxazole and rifampicin may be potential causes.

Acneiform eruptions

Skin changes resembling acne vulgaris occur with several drugs: corticosteroids (both topical and systemic), adrenocorticotrophic hormone, androgenic drugs in women, lithium and iodides. The changes are usually on the face and upper trunk and tend to be monomorphic, consisting largely of papulopustules. There are seldom comedones present.

Some drugs also exacerbate pre-existing acne (see below).

Hair abnormalities

As discussed in Chapter 13, drugs may be responsible for hair loss or excessive hair growth.

Cytotoxics are the drugs which most commonly cause hair loss, but anticoagulants, antithyroid drugs and retinoids may also be responsible. Increased hair growth in a secondary sexual distribution in females occurs with steroids and agents with androgenic properties. More generalized hypertrichosis is seen in patients treated with minoxidil, cyclosporin A, diazoxide, phenytoin and penicillamine.

Pigmentary changes

Several drugs cause hyperpigmentation. Clofazimine, an agent used in the treatment of leprosy, produces a highly characteristic generalized reddish brown hue. Mepacrine and β-carotene both stain the skin yellow. Rather bizarre hyperpigmentation can result from the use of chloroquine and prolonged ingestion of high dose minocycline. Chlorpromazine may induce a widespread purplish colour. Silver may be deposited in the skin following the use of anti-smoking lozenges containing silver salts. Amiodarone is another cause of drug-induced pigmentation, usually on the face. Oestrogens can precipitate or exaggerate chloasma.

Bullous reactions

Bullae may arise on fixed drug eruptions (see above). Drugs may also induce pemphigus and pemphigoid (see Chapter 14). Drugs may exacerbate blistering in porphyria cutanea tarda (see below). A dramatic phototoxic reaction with bulla formation on the lower legs is occasionally seen in patients who have taken nalidixic acid. Sedatives such as barbiturates may cause bullae on pressure points, usually in patients who have been unconscious because of an overdose.

Photosensitivity

Many drugs cause photosensitivity and there are three main types of reaction: exacerbation of underlying disease (see below); direct phototoxic reaction; or photoallergic reaction. In phototoxic reactions, the dose of the drug and the intensity of the UV exposure may both be important. If critical dose levels are not reached the reaction may not develop. This can lead to diagnostic confusion if the drug has been taken on a number of occasions.

Patients usually complain that exposure to the sun initially causes a burning sensation. This is then followed by erythema, swelling and, later, frankly eczematous changes. The affected areas are, of course, predominantly light-exposed (Fig. 21.4). Drugs frequently incriminated include phenothiazines, sulphonamides, tetracyclines and thiazides. Demethylchlortetracycline can cause photo-onycholysis. Bullae which are due to nalidixic acid have been mentioned above.

Lupus erythematosus-like syndrome

A rare but important drug reaction is the induction of a syndrome closely resembling systemic lupus erythematosus. There is a long list of agents that

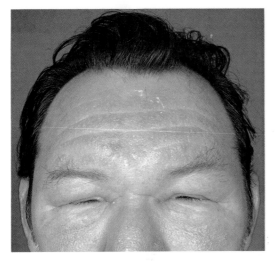

Fig. 21.4. Photosensitivity to sulphonamide.

have been incriminated, including hydralazine, isoniazid, penicillin, procaineamide and griseofulvin.

Exacerbation of pre-existing disease

It is important to recognize that some drugs may produce a deterioration in certain skin disorders. Notable examples are:

1 *Acne* This may be exacerbated by androgenic drugs (e.g. danazol, stanozolol), oral contraceptives and corticosteroids.

2 *Porphyrias* The clinical features, including cutaneous photosensitivity, may be worsened by drug ingestion, particularly barbiturates and oestrogens.

3 *Psoriasis* This may be made worse by treatment with lithium.

4 *Systemic lupus erythematosus* The use of penicillin and sulphonamides may be associated with a deterioration.

Conclusion

If you use all the clinical information at your disposal, i.e.:

A good history

A careful examination

Elimination of other skin diseases

Recognition of a rash as a possible drug reaction

Recognition of the type of clinical reaction pattern

Matching the reaction with the most likely offending agent.

Tests, where appropriate (possibly including a challenge).

It is often possible to come to a reasonable conclusion in many instances.

Chapter 22
Treatment of Skin Disease

If it's dry, wet it. If it's wet, dry it. Congratulations, you are now a dermatologist!
(Anonymous)

The above witticism is oft-quoted by non-dermatologists as an assessment of the scope of dermatological therapeutics. An alternative calumny relates to a dermatologist murmuring unintelligible Latin names as a diagnosis, and then prescribing a certain well-known fluorinated topical steroid, for everything. Apart from being deeply offensive to sensitive skin doctors, both these quips are far from the truth, as dermatologists have an enormous therapeutic armamentarium at their disposal. In days of yore, it must be admitted, many of the available topical therapies were somewhat cosmetically unacceptable and often malodorous—if the skin disease did not render the patient a social pariah, the treatment could be relied upon to do so. However, in recent years, scientific and technological advances have meant that most topical therapies are not only more effective than of old, but also cosmetically much more acceptable.

We have already dealt with the treatment of individual disorders in the preceding chapters, so this chapter is designed to provide an overview of the principles of topical therapy.

The ideal topical preparation for the management of skin disease would be one which penetrates well, but whose activity remains entirely localized within the skin, thus avoiding potential problems from systemic effects. In practice this is extremely difficult to achieve, and any agent which penetrates the stratum corneum to act on the epidermis and dermis is going to be absorbed to some extent.

Every topical preparation consists of an active ingredient or ingredients, and a material in which this is suspended—a so-called base. The active ingredients and the base must be compatible. There is no point in discovering a new base which penetrates the skin like a hot knife through butter if it completely inactivates everything suspended in it. As mentioned in Chapter 1 the stratum corneum forms an efficient barrier to penetration of externally applied materials, and this includes therapeutic agents. To aid penetration of topically applied drugs, we can attempt to break down the barrier function of the stratum corneum. Hydration of the stratum corneum impairs its barrier function, and this can be achieved by occlusion of the skin. For example, penetration of a topical steroid may be markedly enhanced by occluding an area of skin with polythene. Unfortunately, if large areas of skin are occluded in this way the amount of steroids absorbed will be sufficient to produce significant systemic effects. Bases containing urea also hydrate the stratum corneum and enhance penetration of their active ingredients. Dimethyl sulphoxide (DMSO) is a solvent which has a remarkable ability to penetrate skin extremely rapidly and is used as a vehicle for the antiviral agent idoxuridine in the treatment of herpes simplex and shingles.

Bases

Bases include creams, oily creams, ointments, lotions, gels, and pastes. A cream is an oil-in-water emulsion which is relatively non-greasy and has only limited emollient activity. Creams are cosmetically acceptable and can be used to treat either moist or dry skin conditions. Oily creams are water-in-oil emulsions which combine good emollient properties with cosmetic acceptability and are therefore of benefit in dry skin conditions. Ointments are greasy preparations which have emollient and occlusive properties. The occlusive effect of an ointment results in hydration of the stratum corneum and enhanced penetration of any active ingredient the ointment might contain. The benefits of ointments are offset by lack of cosmetic acceptability in use. Ointments are messy and stick to clothing. If used on the hands they transfer to everything touched—an obvious disadvantage in someone employed in clerical work. Lotions are fluid preparations which have a cooling effect resulting from evaporation. They are useful in the management of moist, exudative skin lesions, and also in dermatoses affecting the scalp. Clear, non-greasy gels are designed for use on hairy parts of the body, where they are cosmetically acceptable. Pastes are powders, usually mixed with soft paraffin, and are protective—for example in the prevention of maceration of the skin around a discharging ulcer.

The choice of a particular base should be determined by the type of skin problem and the sites affected. It is, for example, wholly inappropriate to prescribe a steroid ointment for daytime use on the scalp—unless the patient is bald or works a night-shift—because it is far too messy. A gel or lotion preparation should be used on the scalp. Similarly, a lotion preparation is not the correct base to use on ichthyotic skin, where an oily cream or ointment base is much more appropriate.

Bases are not usually simple substances, but are mixtures of several components, formulated to provide stability and freedom from microbial contamination. Random dilution of a topical preparation will dilute the preservatives in the base and significantly shorten its shelf life. Dermatologists used to prescribe large quantities of diluted topical steroids, all marked with a 'Do not use after . . . 'date—frequently this was 4 weeks before the patient's next appointment. The availability of proprietary topical steroids in a variety of strengths has rendered dilution almost obsolete.

Communication and patient compliance

Most non-topical medication simply involves popping pills of various colours into the mouth at certain times of the day. Good compliance usually means managing to take a q.d.s. regime at least b.d., and at least 3 days of a 7-day course. Topical therapy demands a great deal more of the patient, and the increased effort required of the patient ought to be matched by more precise instructions from the dermatologist. For example, a patient suffering from psoriasis might be given a tar shampoo, a scalp lotion, a mild topical steroid cream to use in the flexures, and a dithranol preparation for short contact therapy to plaques on the trunk and limbs. If that patient has only recently developed psoriasis and is not familiar with the treatment, unless the doctor provides written instructions telling the patient which preparation to use where, the patient may put the dithranol in the flexures, the lotion on the trunk and limbs, and the steroid cream in the scalp. Verbal instructions are not sufficient if multiple topical therapies are prescribed.

Do not expect a patient who departs for work at the crack of dawn to adhere strictly to instructions to wash his hair every morning and use a topical medication twice daily. Modify the treatment schedule to suit the individual. If you are prescribing a preparation which is messy to use and/or malodorous, warn the patient about this. For example, dithranol stains, and benzoyl peroxide bleaches, and lack of prior warning could lead to ruined clothing and bed-sheets.

Quantities prescribed

It is important when prescribing topical therapy to estimate the area to be covered and the frequency of application before assessing the quantity of a topical agent required by the patient. There is little point, for example, in prescribing a 30 g tube of an emollient to be used over the entire body surface after bathing—a repeat prescription would be required after one application, because this is the approximate amount required for a single application over the whole body surface of an adult. Topical therapies are available in a variety of container sizes. You will need to check the available sizes before prescribing, as they vary from product to product. Topical steroids, for example, may be marketed in 5, 15, 25, 30, 50 or 100 g tubes, depending on the manufacturer. Most emollients are available in 50 and 100 g tubes and 500 g tubs or dispensers.

Underprescribing of topical therapy is a common fault, but so also is overprescribing. One does not require 100 g of cream to treat a small patch of eczema on the leg—whether the eczema responds to treatment or not, most of the tube will languish in a drawer or bathroom cabinet until its shelf-life is long expired, or worse still may be inappropriately used by some other member of the family. The overprescribing of large quantities of potent topical steroids is potentially likely to cause problems, and should be avoided.

Topical steroids

At first sight the huge number of available topical steroid preparations may seem bewildering to the uninitiated. In fact, with a little knowledge and experience their use is quite straightforward.

Topical steroids may be divided into several groups according to potency. Hydrocortisone preparations are the weakest of the topical steroids. A few products containing hydrocortisone are more potent because their bases contain urea which enhances penetration of the stratum corneum by the hydrocortisone. Modification of the basic steroid skeleton by fluorination or esterification produces steroids of much greater potency (Table 22.1).

Table 22.1   Topical steroid potency (British National Formulary)

Group	Potency	Examples
IV	Mild	1% hydrocortisone Alclometasone diproprionate (Modrasone)
III	Moderately potent	Clobetasone butyrate (Eumovate) Flurandrenalone (Haelan) Hydrocortisone with urea (Alphaderm)
II	Potent	Betamethasone valerate (Betnovate) Fluocinolone acetonide (Synalar) Fluocinonide (Metosyn) Hydrocortisone butyrate (Locoid)
I	Very potent	Clobetasol propionate (Dermovate) Diflucortolone valerate (Nerisone Forte)

Choice of preparation

The most appropriate topical steroid for a given situation should be determined by the type and severity of the condition being treated, the sites affected, and the age of the patient. It goes without saying that the condition being treated should be steroid-responsive, and that topical steroids must not be used in the treatment of viral, bacterial or fungal infections of the skin. The skin disorders which are steroid-responsive have been delineated in previous chapters, and include various types of eczema, lichen planus, psoriasis of the scalp, flexures, hands and feet, and discoid lupus erythematosus. In general, a severe dermatosis should be treated with a potent steroid, and a mild condition with a weak steroid. In the case of a chronic dermatosis subject to periodic exacerbations a mild–moderate potency steroid can be used when the condition is quiescent, and a potent preparation to control the exacerbations.

There are distinct regional variations in the absorption of topical steroids through the skin and their potential for local adverse effects. These variations are determined by the thickness of the stratum corneum, occlusion, for example in the flexures, and the vascularity of the area. Most facial dermatoses should only be treated with mild topical steroids, although a few conditions such as discoid lupus erythematosus will require potent preparations. Skin disease affecting the axillae, groins and submammary areas should also be treated with mild topical steroids. Conversely, dermatoses of the palms of the hands and soles of the feet, where the stratum corneum is extremely thick, will require potent steroids to produce any benefit.

There is a greater risk of adverse systemic effects from the use of topical steroids in children because of the increased absorption related to a high ratio of skin surface area to body volume, particularly in infants. For this reason only mild topical steroids should be used in small children. The skin of the elderly is thin, and potent steroids will exacerbate this change—their use over protracted periods of time in the elderly should therefore be avoided.

Side-effects

Side-effects are rarely seen following the use of mild topical steroids, but they are encountered more frequently in association with potent topical steroid use. Side-effects may be divided into local, occurring at the site of application of the steroid, and systemic, resulting from percutaneous absorption.

Local

Atrophy of the skin Topical steroids produce dose-related thinning of the dermis. This effect is particularly noticeable in areas where the skin is naturally relatively thin, such as the axillae, medial aspect of the upper arm, groins, and the medial aspect of the thigh. Prominent striae may develop in these areas (Fig. 22.1). On the face, cutaneous thinning and telangiectasis produce prominent erythema.

Peri-oral dermatitis Peri-oral dermatitis is a condition usually seen in young women who have used potent topical steroids on the face for lengthy periods

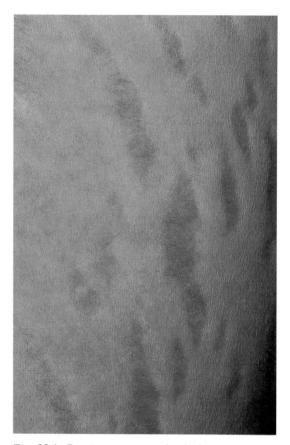

Fig. 22.1. Prominent striae on the thighs.

of time. The eruption consists of small papules and pustules on an erythematous background, and as the name suggests these changes occur around the mouth (Fig. 22.2). In the majority of cases the steroid has been inappropriately prescribed for mild acne on the chin. The history given by patients suffering from peri-oral dermatitis is virtually identical in all cases. Initially the condition for which the steroid was prescribed appears to improve, probably because the vasoconstrictor activity of the steroid reduces erythema, and inflammatory papules become less noticeable. However, stopping treatment results in a rebound flare of the erythema, and the patient therefore considers the treatment is keeping the condition controlled and continues to apply the steroid; she may even increase the frequency of application. Eventually, as the eruption around her mouth becomes more noticeable, she asks her doctor if there is anything 'stronger' which she can use, and is often given a more potent topical steroid, Treatment of peri-oral dermatitis consists of stopping the potent steroid, warning the patient about the rebound flare of erythema which will occur, and prescribing a mild topical steroid for 2–3 weeks to reduce the severity of the flare. In addition, oxytetracycline is of benefit in this condition, although the reason for its efficacy is not understood, and should be given in a dose of 500 mg b.d., gradually reducing over a period of several weeks as the condition improves.

Steroid rosacea Topical steroids will worsen pre-existing rosacea, and can precipitate a rosacea-like eruption.

Infection Staphylococcal folliculitis may occur in areas treated with topical steroids, particularly when ointments or polythene occlusion are used, and the

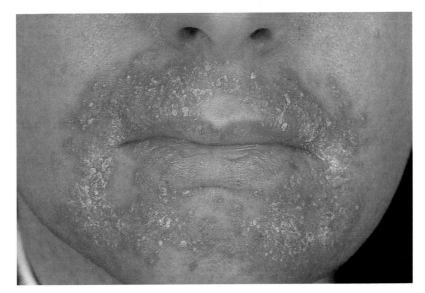

Fig. 22.2. Peri-oral dermatitis.

use of steroids in moist, warm flexural areas may encourage superinfection with *Candida*. Inappropriate use of topical steroids on dermatophyte fungal infections alters the appearance of the eruption, producing so-called 'tinea incognito' (see Chapter 4). Scabies treated with topical steroids becomes extremely florid, with many burrows and a very numerous mite population (see Chapter 5).

Systemic effects

Topical steroids are absorbed through the skin, and excessive use of potent steroids may result in iatrogenic Cushing's syndrome. This problem is rarely encountered nowadays, because those prescribing potent steroids have become more familiar with their potential adverse effects, and restrict the amounts prescribed.

Children are most susceptible than adults to the systemic effects of topical steroids, and growth retardation is an important consequence of the use of long-term potent topical steroid therapy.

Index

dyshidrotic
eczema
palms, fingers
soles.
hi dose topic
steroids
cold compress
? low cobalt
diet,
oxybutynin
(ditropan)